Immunology of Pregnancy

Chemical Immunology and Allergy

Vol. 89

KARGER

Immunology of Pregnancy

Volume Editor

Udo R. Markert *Jena*

16 figures, 2 in color, and 3 tables, 2005

KARGER

Basel · Freiburg · Paris · London · New York ·
Bangalore · Bangkok · Singapore · Tokyo · Sydney

Chemical Immunology and Allergy
Formerly published as 'Progress in Allergy' (Founded 1939),
continued 1990-2002 as 'Chemical Immunology'
Edited by Paul Kallos 1939-1988, Byron H. Waksman 1962–2002

Udo R. Markert
Placenta-Labor
Abteilung für Geburtshilfe
Friederich-Schiller-Universität
D-07740 Jena

Bibliographic Indices. This publication is listed in bibliographic services, including Current Contents® and Index Medicus.

Drug Dosage. The authors and the publisher have exerted every effort to ensure that drug selection and dosage set forth in this text are in accord with current recommendations and practice at the time of publication. However, in view of ongoing research, changes in government regulations, and the constant flow of information relating to drug therapy and drug reactions, the reader is urged to check the package insert for each drug for any change in indications and dosage and for added warnings and precautions. This is particularly important when the recommended agent is a new and/or infrequently employed drug.

www.karger.com
Printed in Switzerland on acid-free paper by Reinhardt Druck, Basel
ISSN 1660–2242
ISBN 3–8055–7970–5

Contents

Preface

This book presents the discipline of immunology which studies a unique physiological phenomenon contradicting many of the generally established rules in the field: immunology of pregnancy. It provides a wide overview of the current research of this topic. Prominent and leading international groups contributed by reviewing the most significant findings in the field.

Pregnancy is the symbiosis of two allogeneic individuals which live in intimate contact. The maternal immune system reacts towards the foreign tissue, but instead of triggering rejection, it tolerates, supports and regulates its development. It controls efficiently and indispensably the formation of the placenta and thereby the development of the embryo and fetus. Many internal and external factors can provoke imbalances of the system, which may result in pregnancy disorders including infertility and abortions.

Leading scientists in the field present the latest findings on physiological mechanisms required for successful pregnancies and the respective pathologies. The regulation of maternal NK cells, T cells and dendritic cells through hormones, cytokines, complement system and HLA as well as other cell-surface molecules are described in detail.

Knowledge of the immunoregulatory processes of pregnancy is necessary to understand and treat a variety of disorders, which may lead to infertility, premature events, preeclamptic diseases and many other problems. The same knowledge can be used to gain insight into distant fields of immunology, where immunomodulatory mechanisms known from pregnancy are involved in pathologies, such as HLA-G or progesterone-induced blocking factor (PIBF) in tumor development, or in therapeutic approaches, such as in posttransplantation or allergy therapies.

This book presents fascinating facets of immunology, which may surprise those readers who are not yet familiar with the immunology of reproduction and which will update the knowledge of specialists.

The general political and public interest in the field is reflected by the establishment and support of a European Network of Excellence entitled EMBIC (Embryo Implantation Control; www.embic.org; 2004–2008), which is strongly supported by the European Union. Several of the authors of this book are partners of the EMBIC.

Udo R. Markert

Market UR (ed): Immunology of Pregnancy.
Chem Immunol Allergy. Basel, Karger, 2005, vol 89, pp 1–2

The 'Hatching' of Reproductive Immunology

Radslav Kinský

Zdar nad Sazavou, Czech Republic

Transplantation immunology has progressed since Paul Bert's experiments on rats in the 19th century regarding the riddle of the mother's acceptance of an antigenically different fetus carrying paternal antigens. The modification of the pregnant female's immune reactivity became a topic developed by several research workers. Vera and Milan Hasek contributed largely to the field during the days and years of 'specific acquired tolerance' in the early 1950s, showing in particular that the pregnant mother was able to reject foreign and even paternal tissue grafts when transplanted to an ectopic site. Furthermore, fetal tissue was sufficiently immunogenic to elicit a rejection reaction when grafted on to a third party or maternal recipient. Therefore, attention was focused on local events linked to the placenta and trophoblast and to the hormonal balance during pregnancy. The long list of lymphokines and cytokines present in the vicinity of the implantation site and the crucial role of NK cells and their respective control represented topics aimed at an explanation of various types of failure of fetal development and abortions. It was soon clear that a large number of conditions and factors were involved in the chain of events during pregnancy, beginning at the early stages (e.g. EPF = early pregnancy factor). However, the lack of even one factor or step can lead to fetal demise. This is often compared to a delicate and complex mechanism in which the removal of a single small part is able to stop the functioning of the whole 'machine'. This was clearly shown in the work of Julia Szekeres-Bartho studying PIBF (progesterone-induced blocking factor). Furthermore, the role of humoral antibodies and suppressor cells linked reproductive immunology to immunological enhancement facilitation. This facet was thoroughly studied by Gérard Chaouat and myself in Guy Voisin's laboratory in Paris. With Gérard Chaouat we further showed the role of anti-idiotypic antibodies and later with Ricardo Margni and Ruben Binaghi the participation of the so-called 'incomplete antibodies', not fixing C and significantly increased during pregnancy mainly in the long-term gravidity of the equine species. Over half a century the working conditions in our laboratories, using various kits of highly specific materials, sophisticated apparatuses with automatic distributors and measurements, have made it possible to shift efforts in the present scientific community from benchwork to the field of invention and intellectual originality. I remember one of Professor Pierre Grabar's remarks stating that when at the end of his career and life he visited modern laboratories with extraordinarily expensive equipment he still thought that the outstanding work achieved by the scientists of his generation with their own hands was mainly possible because they were close to the actual realization of their results.

Radslav Kinský
ZÁMEK c. 13/13
591 02 Zdar nad Sazavou (Czech Republic)

Markert UR (ed): Immunology of Pregnancy.
Chem Immunol Allergy. Basel, Karger, 2005, vol 89, pp 3–9

T Cells in Pregnancy

Marie-Pierre Piccinni

Department of Internal Medicine, Immunoallergology Unit,
University of Florence, Florence, Italy

Abstract

Maternal tolerance of the fetal allograft could be the result of the integration of numerous mechanisms promoted by different cells present in the decidua. Decidual macrophages and dendritic cells, which are found in close association with T lymphocytes are the most potent activators of T lymphocyte responses and could play a sentinel function for the immune system, initiating antigen-specific T cell responses to fetal antigens. T cell cytokines produced in response to fetal molecules could have a role in the maintenance or in the failure of pregnancy. The levels of LIF, IL-4, IL-10 and M-CSF produced by decidual T cells of women suffering from unexplained spontaneous abortion are lower than those of normal pregnant women indicating that these cytokines may contribute to the maintenance of pregnancy. T cells from the cumulus oophorus surrounding the preimplantation embryo produce LIF and IL-4. These findings suggest that cytokines produced by maternal T cells create a suitable microenvironment for preimplantation embryo development and maintenance of pregnancy. T cell cytokine profile could be modulated by the hormones present in the microenvironment of T cells: high doses of progesterone present at fetomaternal interface and in the cumulus induce the production of IL-4 and LIF, whereas relaxin induces IFN-γ production.

Introduction

In pregnancy, the embryo implants into the specialized mucosal wall of the uterus (decidua) and the placenta starts to form. Trophoblast invades into the uterine mucosa in order to open up maternal uterine arteries to ensure an adequate supply of blood to the developing fetus. The uterine mucosa differentiates in preparation for implantation. One of the changes that takes place is the appearance in the endometrium of a large number of maternal leukocytes in the final part of the menstrual cycle. If pregnancy ensues, these leukocytes continue to increase in number and are found in close contact with trophoblast. Natural killer (NK) cells, macrophages and T cells are the most abundant immunocytes present in the decidua, whereas B cells are virtually absent. It is apparent that immunological mechanism may play an important role in pregnancy. We outline below the possible roles of T cells in successful pregnancy, pregnancy failure and preimplantation embryo development.

Decidual T Cells

In early pregnancy, the T cells comprise 10–20% of the leukocytes in the uterine mucosa. The relative number of T cells is greater during implantation. Many years ago, a role of T cells in the development of the placenta and in the fetal survival was suggested. The injection of anti-T cell antibodies in MRL-lpr/lpr homologous mice, which exhibit excessive T cell proliferation and large placentas, reduced placental parameters to normal [1]. In normal mice, the same treatment decreased placental size and in some strain combinations caused fetal resorption [1].

Inasmuch as many T cell effects are mediated via the production of cytokines, the type of cytokines produced could influence the maintenance of the fetoplacental unit. The human CD4+ T cells can be classified on the basis of their pattern of cytokine production [2, 3]. Type 1 CD4+ T cells (Th1) produce interleukin (IL)-2, tumor necrosis factor-β and interferon (IFN)-γ and are the main effectors of phagocyte-mediated host defense, which is highly protective against infections sustained by intracellular parasites [2, 3]. On the other hand, type 2 CD4+ T cells (Th2) produce IL-4, which stimulate IgE and IgG1 antibody production, IL-5 (promoting the growth and the differentiation of eosinophils), IL-13 and IL-10 which together with IL-4 inhibit several macrophage functions. The Th2 cell is mainly responsible for phagocyte-independent host defense, e.g. against certain nematodes [2, 3].

The maternal decidua, which is in direct contact with the trophoblast, contains macrophages, dentritic cells and T lymphocytes. These cell types are potentially able to promote the rejection of fetal allograft, which is first mediated by the recognition of paternal MHC antigens by the antigen-presenting cells (dendritic cells and macrophages) and then by the activity of effector T cells via the release of various cytokines. Therefore, changes in the recognition mechanisms and/or in the pattern of cytokines produced by the activated T cells may play an important role in the immunological tolerance of the conceptus during successful pregnancy, as well as in its premature rejection. It appears that some Th1-dependent effector mechanisms play a central role in acute allograft rejection. Proteins and/or transcripts for intragraft IL-2,

IFN-γ and the cytotoxic T lymphocytes-specific marker, granzyme B, have consistently been detected in rejecting allografts [4, 5]. Several in vivo studies that examined the pattern of cytokine expression during tolerance induction have consistently shown a dramatic decrease in the expression of IL-2 and IFN-γ, while increased levels of IL-4 and IL-10 transcripts are manifest [4, 5]. This has suggested, maybe in a simplistic way, that Th1-type cytokines, that promote allograft rejection [4, 5], may compromise pregnancy, whereas the Th2-type cytokines, inhibiting the Th1 responses, promote allograft tolerance and therefore may improve fetal survival.

Th1- and Th2-type cytokines produced by maternal T lymphocytes present at fetomaternal interface seem to play a role in the development of pregnancy. In mice, it has been reported that IL-4, IL-5 and IL-10 are detectable at the fetomaternal interface throughout the period of gestation, whereas IFN-γ is transient, being detectable only in the first period [6, 7]. In humans, studies of pathological conditions can shed light on the normal situation in the uterus. In women suffering from unexplained recurrent abortion with histories of at least 3 prior first-trimester spontaneous abortions, which cannot be explained on the basis of the conventional criteria, a role of the detrimental immune system has been suggested. Indeed, we have shown a defect of IL-4 production by both decidual CD4+ and CD8+ T cells and a defect of IL-10 and M-CSF by decidual CD4+ T cells of women suffering from unexplained recurrent abortion undergoing a spontaneous abortion in comparison with the decidual T cells of women with a normal pregnancy undergoing a voluntary abortion [8, 9]. Accordingly, very recently in women with unexplained recurrent abortion with normal chromosomal content a decrease of CD4+ and CD8+ T cells expressing CRTH2, a marker of Th2 and Tc2 cells, at the site of implantation, has been observed [10]. Therefore, in humans at the fetomaternal interface the success of pregnancy seems to be associated with the production of IL-4, IL-10 and M-CSF by T cells [8, 9, 11]. The defect in IL-10 production by decidual T cells of women suffering from unexplained recurrent abortion is consistent with the results obtained in abortion-prone CBA × DBA/2 mice. These mice have placentas deficient in IL-10 and intraperitoneal injection of IL-10 reduces fetal loss to a normal level [12]. Interestingly, the levels of IFN-γ produced by decidual T cells of women with unexplained recurrent abortion and normal pregnancy did not differ. Therefore, we did not find an increased production of IFN-γ by decidual T cells during the spontaneous abortion, as could be expected because of the potential role of Th1-type cytokines on allograft rejection.

Leukemia inhibitory factor (LIF) is an endometrial requirement for implantation and embryo development, inasmuch as female mice lacking a functional LIF gene are fertile but their blastocysts fail to implant and do not develop unless the blastocysts are transferred to wild-type pseudopregnant recipients or the animals are treated locally with LIF [13]. We have seen that LIF known to be produced by endometrial epithelial cells and NK cell is also produced by T cells and mainly by Th2-like cells [8]. Finally, we have found not only a defective production of IL-4 and IL-10 in decidual T cells of women suffering from unexplained recurrent abortion, but also a defective production of LIF by these cells [8]. All these results suggest that T cell LIF, M-CSF and Th2-type cytokine production at the fetomaternal interface could contribute to the development of pregnancy. The relative contribution of LIF produced by T cells compared with the contribution of LIF produced by endometrium epithelial cells or NK cells is not clear. Recently, it has been reported that in the decidua there is a strong LIF mRNA expression among the CD45+ leukocytes. Little or no expression of LIF mRNA was seen in the glandular epithelium of the decidua, even though adjacent CD45+ leukocytes were strongly positive. Interestingly, in nonpregnant endometrium, the glandular epithelium expresses abundant LIF mRNA with little apparent expression by leukocytes [14]. Therefore, LIF expression by glandular epithelium is dramatically downregulated after implantation, whereas expression by leukocytes is upregulated in the decidua. The authors assigned most of the LIF expression to NK cells that represent 70% of the leukocytes present in the decidua. However, decidual NK cells (the apparent source) purified and cultured alone did not produce LIF even if these cells were stimulated by exogenous IL-2, IL-1β or IFN-γ [14]. Therefore, it seems that the production of LIF protein in the deciduas during pregnancy could be predominantly assigned to the T cells.

A reduced production of Th2-type cytokines, LIF and M-CSF at the fetomaternal interface in women suffering from unexplained recurrent abortion has not been found at the level of peripheral blood, suggesting that this is not an inherent feature of T cells, but rather a microenvironmentally oriented alteration. We wonder what are the factors present in the microenvironment of the T cells that could be responsible for the cytokine profile of the T cells in unexplained recurrent abortion and in successful pregnancy. The cytokine profile of T cells in pregnancy could be influenced by hormones. Progesterone, at concentrations comparable to those present at the maternofetal interface during pregnancy, is a potent inducer of the production of Th2-type cytokines (i.e. IL-4 and IL-5) [12], but also a potent inducer of LIF and M-CSF production by T cells. The productions of M-CSF and LIF induced by progesterone are mediated by IL-4 [8, 11, 15–17]. Moreover, relaxin, a polypeptide hormone predominantly produced by the corpus luteum and decidua during pregnancy, favors the development of T cells producing IFN-γ, without exerting any effect on the production of IL-4 [18]. 17β-Estradiol and hCG have no effect on the T cell differentiation into Th1 or Th2 cells [15]. Therefore, hormonal influences seem to play a critical role in determining the T cell cytokine pattern at the fetomaternal interface [8, 11, 15–18].

Our results suggest a hormone-cytokine-T cell network at the fetomaternal interface. Progesterone, present at a high level at the fetomaternal interface, may be at least in part responsible for a Th2 switch at the fetomaternal interface. IL-4 produced by the Th2 cells can in turn promote the development of T cells producing LIF and M-CSF, which seem to be important for embryo implantation and development. Both IL-4 and IL-10 can inhibit the development and function of Th1 cells and macrophages, thus preventing the allograft rejection. Moreover, both IL-10- and IL-4-promoting progesterone production by luteal cells derived from corpora lutea of early pregnancy [19] could amplify this possible mechanism. A defect in the integrity of this network may result in fetal loss. Obviously, the possibility that functional changes in T cells are the result rather than the cause of pregnancy failure cannot be excluded. Even in this case, however, T cell functional alterations may aggravate the situation and accelerate the rejection.

Cumulus Oophorus T Cells

In most mammals, T cells are not confined exclusively to the uterus. We detected T cells in the large and expanded mass of cells, called cumulus oophorus, which surrounds the oocyte during ovulation. Clusters of these cells progressively detach, but variable numbers of cells remain around the egg for the first 72 h before the implantation of the blastocyst in the uterus [20]. We have detected both macrophages and CD4+ T cells in all cumuli from women suffering from blocked fallopian tubes, who underwent an in vitro fertilization program. However, only very few NK cells have been found occasionally [21]. These cumulus T cells produce higher levels of IL-4 and LIF than the T cells of peripheral blood or ovary specimens isolated from the same women. Of note, although T cells from the cumulus oophorus were derived from the ovary, they produced higher levels of IL-4 and lower levels of IL-10 than T cells from biopsy specimens of the ovaries. This finding demonstrates that T cells present in the cumulus oophorus are different from other T cells present in the ovary and suggests the existence of a peculiar microenvironmental orientation for cumulus T cells [21]. As was suggested for decidua, hormones can modulate the cytokine profile of the cumulus oophorus T cells. Very high levels of progesterone found in the culture medium of human cumulus-oocyte/fertilized egg complexes [22], produced by cumulus luteal cells, may favor IL-4 production by T cells, which in turn can produce LIF. The physiological meaning of LIF and IL-4 production by T cells present in the cumulus oophorus is unclear and may only be an object of speculation. The treatment with LIF enhances the in vitro growth and development of murine [23], bovine [24] and ovine [25] embryos, suggesting that LIF and probably other cytokines acting in concert with LIF are required to create a suitable microenvironment for the early embryo development.

Conclusion

T cells could play a role in embryo development and implantation and in the maternal tolerance towards the fetus. The T cells could work in parallel with NK cells, macrophages and/or dendritic cells restraining or increasing the effects of these cells. The integration of numerous mechanisms of various origins could be responsible for the maternal tolerance towards the fetus [26–28].

Acknowledgments

The author of this manuscript is member of an European Network of Excellence, entitled 'EMBIC' (Embryo Implantation Control), supported by the European Union (contract no. 512040).

References

1 Chaouat G, Menu E, Athanassakis I, Wegmann TG: Maternal T cells regulate placental size and fetal survival. Reg Immunol 1988;1:143–148.
2 Mosmann TR, Coffman RL: Th1 and Th2 cells: Different patterns of lymphokine secretion lead to different functional properties. Annu Rev Immunol 1989;7:145–173.
3 Romagnani S: Human Th1 and Th2: Doubt no more. Immunol Today 1991;12:256–257.
4 Suthanthiran M, Strom TB: Immunobiology and immunopharmacology of organ allograft rejection. J Clin Immunol 1995;15:161–171.
5 Nickerson P, Steurer W, Steiger J, Zheng X, Steele AW, Strom TB: Cytokines and the Th1/Th2 paradigm in transplantation. Curr Opin Immunol 1994;6:757–764.
6 Lin H, Mosmann TR, Guilbert L, Tuntipopipat S, Wegmann TG: Synthesis of T helper 2-type cytokines at maternal-fetal interface. J Immunol 1993;151:4562–4573.
7 Wegmann TG, Lin H, Guilbert L, Mossmann TR: Bidirectional cytokine interactions in the maternal-fetal relationship: Is successful pregnancy a Th2 phenomenon? Immunol Today 1993;14:353–356.
8 Piccinni M-P, Beloni L, Livi C, Maggi E, Scarselli GF, Romagnani S: Defective production of both leukemia inhibitory factor and type 2 T-helper cytokines by decidual T cells in unexplained recurrent abortions. Nat Med 1998;4:1020–1024.
9 Piccinni M-P, Beloni L, Livi C, Maggi E, Scarselli GF, Romagnani S: The maintenance of pregnancy is associated with predominance of Th2 type-cytokines; in Colarcurci N, Cardone A (eds): The Embryo from Gametogenesis to Implantation. Naples, Giuseppe Nicola editor, 1998, pp 177–180.
10 Michita T, Sakai M, Miyazaki S, Ogasawara MS, Suzumori K, Aoki K, Nagata K, Saito S: Decrease of T helper 2 and T cytotoxic 2 cells at implantation sites occurs in unexplained recurrent abortion with normal chromosomal content. Hum Reprod 2003;18:1523–1528.
11 Piccinni M-P, Scaletti C, Vultaggio A, Maggi E, Romagnani S: Defective production of LIF, M-CSF and Th2-type cytokines by T cells at fetomaternal interface is associated with pregnancy loss. J Reprod Immunol 2001;52:35–43.

12 Chaouat G, Assal-Meliani A, Martal J, Raghupathy R, Elliott J, Mosmann T, Wegmann TG: IL-10 prevents naturally occurring fetal loss in the CBA × DBA/2 mating combination and local defect in IL-10 production in this abortion-prone combination is corrected by in vivo injection of IFN τ. J Immunol 1995;154:4261–4268.
13 Stewart CL, Kaspar P, Brunet LJ, Bhatt H, Gadi I, Kontgen F, Abbondanzo SJ: Blastocyst implantation depends on maternal expression of leukemia inhibitory factor. Nature 1992;359:76–79.
14 Sharkey AM, King A, Clark DE, Burrows TD, Jokhi PP, Charnock-Jones DS, Loke YW, Smith SK: Localization of leukemia inhibitory factor and its receptor in human placenta throughout pregnancy. Biol Reprod 1999;60:335–364.
15 Piccinni M-P, Giudizi MG, Biagiotti R, Beloni L, Giannarini L, Sampognaro S, Parronchi P, Manetti R, Livi C, Romagnani S, Maggi E: Progesterone favors the development of human T helper cells producing Th2-type cytokines and promotes both IL-4 production and membrane CD30 expression in established Th1 cell clones. J Immunol 1995;155:128–133.
16 Piccinni M-P, Maggi E, Romagnani S: Role of hormone-controlled T-cell cytokines in the maintenance of pregnancy. Biochem Soc Trans 2000;28:212–215.
17 Piccinni M-P, Scaletti C, Maggi E, Romagnani S: Role of hormone-controlled Th1- and Th2-type cytokines in successful pregnancy. J Neuroimmunol 2000;109:30–33.
18 Piccinni M-P, Bani D, Beloni L, Manuelli C, Mavilia C, Vocioni F, Bigazzi M, Bani Sacchi T, Romagnani S, Maggi E: Relaxin favors the development of activated human T cells into Th1-like effectors. Eur J Immunol 1999;29:2241–2247.
19 Hashii K, Fujiwara H, Yoshioka S, Kataoka N, Yamada S, Hirano T, Mori T, Fujii S, Maeda M: Peripheral blood mononuclear cells stimulate progesterone production by luteal cells derived from pregnant and non-pregnant women: Possible involvement of interleukin-4 and interleukin-10 in corpus luteum function and differentiation. Hum Reprod 1998;13:2738–2744.
20 Pereda J, Coppo M: An electron microscopic study of sperm penetration into the human egg investments. Anat Embryol 1985;173:247–252.
21 Piccinni M-P, Scaletti C, Mavilia C, Lazzeri E, Romagnani P, Natali I, Pellegrini S, Livi C, Romagnani S, Maggi E: Production of IL-4 and leukemia inhibitory factor by T cells of the cumulus oophorus: A favorable microenvironment for pre-implantation embryo development. Eur J Immunol 2001;31:2431–2437.
22 Laufer N, DeCherney AH, Haseltine FP, Rehrman HR: Steroid secretion by human egg-corona cumulus complexin culture. J Clin Endocrinol Metab 1984;58:1153–1157.
23 Lavranos TC, Rathjen PD, Seamark RF: Trophic effects of myeloid leukemia inhibitory factor (LIF) on mouse embryos. J Reprod Fertil 1995;105:331–338.
24 Funston RN, Nauta WJ, Seidel GE: Culture of bovine embryos in buffalo rat liver cell-conditioned media or with leukemia inhibitory factor. J Anim Sci 1997;75:1332–1336.
25 Fry RC, Batt PA, Fairclough RJ, Parr RA: Human inhibitory factor improves the viability of cultured ovine embryos. Biol Reprod 1995;46:470–474.
26 Piccinni M-P: Role of immune cells in pregnancy. Autoimmunity 2003;36:1–4.
27 Piccinni M-P, Romagnani S: Regulation of fetal allograft survival by hormone-controlled Th1- and Th2-type cytokines. Immunol Res 1996;15:141–150.
28 Piccinni M-P: Cell cytokines in pregnancy. Am J Reprod Immunol 2002;47:1–6.

Dr. Marie-Pierre Piccinni
Dipartimento di Medicina Interna, Sezione di Immunoallergologia
Viale Morgagni, 85, IT–50134 Firenze (Italy)
Tel. +39 055 4271499, Fax +39 055 4271500
E-Mail mppiccinni@hotmail.com

Markert UR (ed): Immunology of Pregnancy.
Chem Immunol Allergy. Basel, Karger, 2005, vol 89, pp 10–25

Physiological Role of IL-15 and IL-18 at the Maternal-Fetal Interface

Gordana Laskarin[a], *Natasa Strbo*[a], *Tatjana Bogovic Crncic*[a], *Koraljka Juretic*[a], *Nathalie Ledee Bataille*[b], *Gerard Chaouat*[b], *Daniel Rukavina*[a]

[a]Department of Physiology and Immunology, Medical Faculty, University of Rijeka, Rijeka, Croatia; [b]U131 INSERM, Hospital Antoine Béclère, Clamart, France

Abstract

We review recent studies of two cytokines IL-15 and IL-18, showing that they are the critical cytokines controlling uterine NK cell cytokine production and cytolytic potential. Further, IL-15 has been implicated in differentiation and proliferation of uterine NK cells, while IL-18 enhanced innate immunity and both Th1- and Th2-driven immune responses depending on the cytokine milieu. We addressed the possible role of these two cytokines in induction of the IFN-γ production as a key molecule in vascular remodeling during early pregnancy.

Interleukin 15

Distribution of IL-15 and IL-15R at the Maternal-Fetal Interface

IL-15 is a four α-helical cytokine (14–15 kDa) that was first identified as a T cell growth factor (IL-T) and was subsequently found to be also essential for NK cell development [1–4]. Although IL-2 and IL-15 have numerous overlapping activities on cells of the immune system, the differential expression of these cytokines within tissues and by various cell types suggests that they may perform at least partially distinct physiological functions. While IL-15 is expressed more broadly in a wide variety of tissues (including placenta) and cells, IL-2 is produced only by activated T cells and LPS-activated dendritic cells [1, 5, 6]. As IL-2 has been detected only in a few samples of isolated decidual T and NK cells by using nested RT-PCR [7], IL-15, therefore, seems likely to provide an important regulatory role for decidual NK cells in vivo.

To mediate its effects, IL-15 interacts with a heterotrimeric receptor that consists of the β and γ subunits of IL-2R, as well as a specific, high-affinity IL-15 binding subunit, which is designated IL-15Rα [8, 9]. IL-2/IL-15Rβ is expressed constitutively by NK cells and to a lesser extent by monocytes and CD8 cells [10, 11]. Expression of the IL-2Rβ by decidual NK cells has previously been reported by many investigators [12–15] as well as the expression of the IL-2Rγ by these cells [14, 15]. IL-15Rα has a wide cellular and tissue distribution [16] including placenta [1]. Its expression is observed in T and B cells, macrophages, in thymic and bone marrow stromal cell lines [17] and recently on purified decidual CD56+ cells [15]. Thus the widespread distribution of IL-15Rα, IL-2/IL-15Rβ and γ_c elements of the IL-15R system is one of the mechanisms underlying the pleiotropy of IL-15.

The murine uterus initiates transcription of IL-15 following onset of decidualization until gestation day 11, when it is lost [18]. Both IL-15 mRNA and protein were demonstrated in the human nonpregnant endometrium, decidua and placenta [15, 18–20]. Moreover IL-15 was detected in uterine macrophages, stromal cells, amnion, and chorion [15, 18, 21] (fig. 1). Kitaya et al. [20] documented that IL-15 protein was localized in glandular epithelial cells and stroma of human endometrium during the late cycle with the most prominent expression in perivascular cells surrounding the decidual spiral arteries. Expression of IL-15 during the early pregnancy is most prominent in endothelial cells of spiral arteries [20]. IL-15 expression was shown to peak in the mid- to late-secretory phase of the normal human menstruation and was upregulated during progesterone-induced decidualization [19]. Progesterone is a potent inducer of IL-15 mRNA expression as well as IL-15 protein secretion in human endometrial stromal cells in vitro [22]. When progesterone levels drop either premenstrually or as a result of a failing pregnancy, the first obvious morphological manifestation is apoptosis of the NK cells which could be the result of a decreasing level of IL-15 [23]. Recently, microarrays have provided expression profiling for endometrium from women with and free from endometriosis during the window of implantation [24]. IL-15 was a candidate gene upregulated during the normal window of implantation but significantly decreased in women with endometriosis [24]. However, exaggerated inflammatory responses may perturb the integrity of endometrial function and lead to pathological conditions. Endometria of women with unexplained recurrent spontaneous abortion express elevated levels of IL-15 compared to control endometrium [25]. Therefore, negative regulators are required to control IL-15 induction associated with disease such as unexplained recurrent spontaneous abortion. Recently, IL-1β has been proposed as one of the negative regulators of IL-15 expression [26].

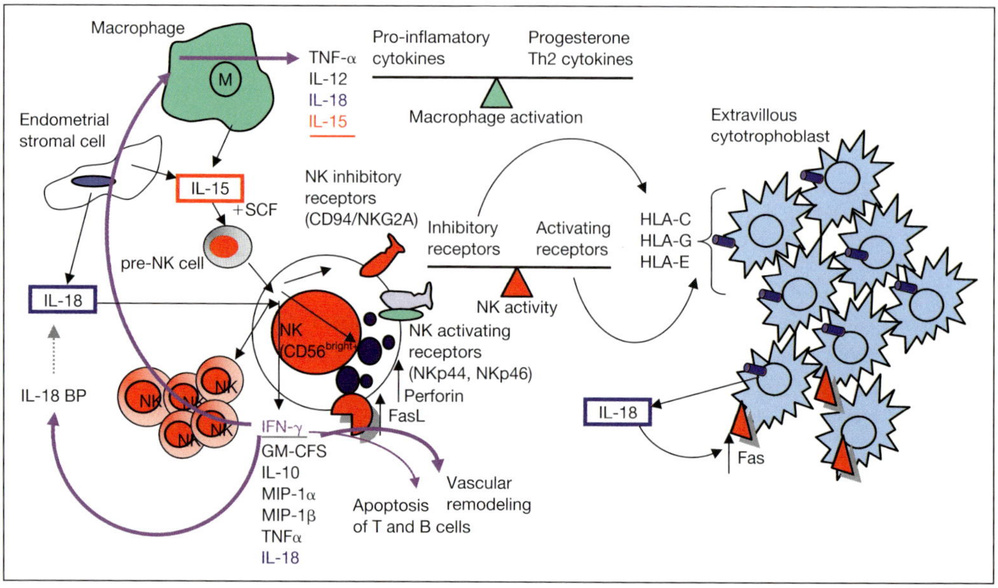

Fig. 1. Biological significance of IL-15 and IL-18 at the maternal-fetal interface. IL-15, mainly produced by decidual macrophages (M) and endometrial stromal cells, together with SCF is involved in maturation of pre-NK cells into CD56bright+ uNK cells. IL-15Rαβγ constitutively expressed on uNK cells binds IL-15 and has been involved in the activation of uNK cells. IL-15 induces uNK proliferation, cytokine production (IFN-γ, GM-CSF, MIP-1α, MIP-1β, TNF-α and IL-18), upregulation of cytolytic mediators (perforin and FasL) and NK receptors (activating: NKp44, NKp46 as well as inhibitory: CD94/NKG2-A). Three MHC class I molecules are expressed by extravillous trophoblast cells (HLA-C, HLA-E and HLA-G) and interact with inhibitory and activating NK receptors. IL-18 at the maternal-fetal interface is produced by endometrial stromal cells, activated macrophages and giant extravillous trophoblast. IL-18 induces perforin expression on uNK cells. IL-18 through IL-18R, constitutively expressed on NK cells and syncytiotrophoblast, and induction of Fas expression on extravillous cytotrophoblast could be involved in the regulation of trophoblast invasion. IFN-γ plays a key role in vascular remodeling, apoptosis of T and B cells and could be induced in uNK cells by IL-15 and IL-18. IFN-γ produced by uNK cells could enhance IL-18BP which decreases proinflammatory activity of IL-18. On the other hand, IFN-γ-stimulated macrophages produce proinflammatory cytokines (TNFα, IL-12, IL-18 and IL-15), which in turn could further augment NK activation. Thus, macrophage-derived IL-15 production should be tightly regulated by Th2 cytokines and progesterone.

Influence of IL-15 on Cytokine Production

Most reports support the classification of IL-15 as a proinflammatory type 1 cytokine [27, 28], whereas a few have considered IL-15 as a costimulatory of type 2 cytokines [29–31] (fig. 1). IL-15 acts in concert with IL-12 to induce the macrophage-activating factors IFN-γ and tumor necrosis factor

(TNF)-α [32, 33] whereas IL-15 alone appears to be a potent stimulus for GM-CSF production [32, 34] by resting CD56 human and murine NK cells [1]. Interestingly, human CD56bright NK cells stimulated with IL-15 plus IL-12 produce approximately 10-fold greater amounts of IFN-γ, TNF-α, and GM-CSF protein compared with an equal number of CD56dim NK cells [34]. Since IL-15 acts as a costimulator of IFN-γ production by NK cells, it may therefore be essential in the control of proinflammatory environment at the implantation site. NK cells also produce the C-C chemokines macrophage inflammatory protein (MIP)-1α and MIP-1β after stimulation with IL-15, which is augmented with the addition of IL-12 [33, 35]. Because C-C chemokines also serve as chemoattractants for NK cells [36], IL-15/IL-12-induced MIP-1α and MIP-1β production may be one mechanism for proper trafficking of additional NK cells to the site of implantation. In addition, chemokine production may have implications in the interactions between macrophages and NK cells, as MIP-1α has been shown to potentiate IFN-γ-inducible secretion of inflammatory cytokines by macrophages [37].

IL-15 is reported to be essential for type 2 cytokine production by NK cells [38]. Stimulation of uterine NK (uNK) cells with IL-2 and IL-15 induced IFN-γ and IL-10 production [39]. IFN-γ production by uNK cell clones was completely inhibited by TGF-β [40]. This suggests that NK cell cytokine production may be governed in part by the monokine IL-15 milieu induced during the early implantation.

Influence of IL-15 on Cytolytic Potential

IL-15 is a cytokine having biological properties similar to those of IL-2 [1, 32]. One such attribute of IL-15 is the ability to generate lymphokine-activated killers from NK cells [1, 2, 32]. IL-15 was found to activate cytotoxicity and antibody-dependent cellular cytotoxicity by sorted CD56bright and CD56dim human NK cell subsets [32]. IL-15 and IL-2 induce nearly identical levels of cytotoxicity, and both depend upon signals through the IL-2/IL-15Rβ [32]. Infection of human PBMCs with herpes viruses resulted in endogenous IL-15-dependent increases in NK cell cytotoxicity, suggesting that IL-15 participates in the normal innate host defense against viral infections [40]. We have found that IL-15 augmented decidual NK cell cytotoxicity against K562 in a dose-dependent manner [41] and Verma et al. [15] reported IL-15-stimulated decidual NK cell killing against JEG-3 but there was little or no cytotoxicity against extravillous trophoblast cells. IL-15 upon binding to IL-2Rβ/IL-15Rα on decidual NK cells leads to the initiation of effector functions including cytotoxicity and secretion of cytokines. Expression of triggering receptors such as NKp44 and NKp46 is under the influence of IL-2 and IL-15 [42, 43] (fig. 1). After their engagement the activation of NK cells occurs. At the same time, it was reported that IL-15 provides an appropriate stimulus to the expression of the inhibitory receptor, CD94/NKG2A, in the process of maturation of NK cells from thymocyte precursors [44] (fig. 1). Relatively little is known about the control of cytotoxic molecule expression by decidual NK cells. Ye et al. [18] demonstrated that IL-15 is involved in regulating the differentiation of granulated metrial gland cells during murine pregnancy. Our preliminary data suggest that IL-15 directly induces upregulation of perforin and FasL mRNA and protein expression on human decidual NK cells [unpubl. data] (fig. 1). We showed an increase of perforin expression in decidual lymphocytes (DL) when activated by IL-2 (1,000 IU/ml) or IL-15 (2 ng/ml) and we proved using inhibitors of granule exocytosis (concanamycin A), a predominant role of perforin-mediated cytotoxicity in unstimulated as well as IL-15-stimulated DL [45, 46]. Further, we found that decidual CD56+ cells, isolated from the suspension of decidual mononuclears following 18 h culture, were equally efficient in lysing NK-susceptible K562 cells as well as the NK-resistant P815 cell line [46]. It is possible that IL-15-activated decidual CD56+ cells, at the maternal-fetal interface, use perforin and Fas/FasL-mediated cytotoxic mechanisms against transformed cells, cells infected with intracellular pathogens or, under specific circumstances, against trophoblast cells.

We demonstrated in vitro that both decidual adherent cell (dAC) and dAC supernatants are responsible for modulation of perforin expression [47, 48]. Further, since these effects could be blocked by anti-IL-15 we proposed that IL-15 has an important role at the maternal-fetal interface in the regulation of perforin expression [47, 49]. Moreover, the membrane-bound IL-15 was observed on decidual CD14+ cells as well as on decidual stromal cells [20]. Depleting decidual macrophages from the suspension of dAC eliminates perforin upregulation, supporting the hypothesis that macrophages and their humoral products (IL-15) have an essential role in perforin expression [48].

Biological Significance of IL-15 at the Maternal-Fetal Interface

With pregnancy changes in stromal and smooth muscle cells of the uterus associated with decidualization elevate IL-15 as well as SCF [15, 50] which both promote survival of pre-NK cells present in and mobilized to the uterus. The SCF receptor c-kit is expressed by blood CD56bright+ cells [51] and also by a proportion of decidual CD56bright cells [52]. This subpopulation may represent the undifferentiated cells capable of a vigorous proliferative response. Since it has been shown that a combination of cytokines including IL-15, SCF, IL-2 and IL-7 [4, 53] induced maturation from an immature (CD34+CD7−) population into CD56+CD3− cells, it is possible that a subpopulation of CD56brightCD16–c-kit+ cells home to the uterine mucosa and differentiate in response to SCF and IL-15 (fig. 1). Recently studies performed by Ashkar et al. [54] clearly demonstrated that IL-15 is absolutely essential for the support of NK cell differentiation in the decidualizing uterus. Analyses of implantation sites in IL-15−/− mice revealed a complete absence of uNK cells as well as a pathology consistent with that seen in other strains severely or totally deficient in uNK cells: unmodified spiral structure of arteries, poor development of decidua and absence of MLAp development within the uterine wall. These features do not compromise fetal viability or postnatal survival [54]. IL-15Rα deficiency is characterized by lymphopenia and NK cell deficiency, again indicating the major role of IL-15 in NK cell development and lymphocyte maintenance [55].

IL-15 has been shown to promote survival of blood NK cells with an increase in *bcl*-2 expression [56]. IL-15 induced the proliferation of CD56bright NK cells in a dose-dependent fashion to a similar extent as IL-2, yet required a nanomolar concentration to activate IL-2/IL-15Rβ for proliferative activity [32]. Proliferation of decidual CD56+ NK cells could be induced by IL-15, also in a dose-dependent manner [15] (fig. 1). A dose of 5 ng/ml produced a maximal proliferative response, which is similar to results reported for blood CD56bright cells [15, 32]. In contrast, the circulating CD56dim cells are reported to respond poorly to IL-15 [32]. Verma et al. [15] have also found that there was a synergistic response when decidual NK cells were cultured with IL-15 (even at suboptimal levels) in contact with a monolayer of irradiated decidual stromal cells, indicating that other factors are responsible for the proliferation in vivo [14]. Other studies support the importance of stromal cells in the proliferation of CD56bright cells. From the pool of CD56+CD3− blood NK cells, only the CD56bright subset was responsible for the expansion mediated by contact with an irradiated murine fibroblast cell line [57]. The close physical association of NK cells to the uterine mucosal stromal cells also suggests a mutual interdependence in vivo. On the other hand, Verma et al. [15] demonstrated that progesterone had an opposite effect on IL-15 production by macrophage-enriched cultures. In contrast to an increased production of IL-15 by stromal cells stimulated with progesterone and PGE_2, progesterone and PGE_2 caused a significant decrease of IL-15 secretion from macrophage-enriched cultures [15]. This could represent an important regulatory mechanism by which progesterone balances innate immune response (fig. 1). It has been demonstrated that autocrine IL-15 regulation of macrophage proinflammatory cytokine production was highly dependent upon the concentrations of IL-15 available to macrophages [58].

Interleukin-18

Distribution of IL-18 and IL-18R Expression at the Maternal-Fetal Interface

IL-18 is an 18-kDa glycoprotein derived by enzymatic cleavage of a 23-kDa precursor, pro-IL-18, by caspase 1 [59]. Pro-IL-18 expression is widespread, including monocyte/macrophages, dendritic cells, Kupffer cells, keratinocytes, articular chondrocytes, synovial fibroblasts and osteoblasts, and within the adrenal cortex and pituitary gland [60]. IL-18 mediates bioactivities through a heterodimeric receptor consisting of α and β chains that are widely expressed on naive T lymphocyte subsets, NK cells, macrophages, neutrophils, and chondrocytes [61]. IL-18Rα, characterized earlier as IL-1R-related protein (IL1Rrp) binds IL-18 at relatively low affinity (in the range of 10^{-8} M) [62]. Generation of IL-18Rα-deficient mice confirmed that this receptor is nevertheless essential for signaling [63]. IL-18Rβ chain, initially termed IL-1 receptor accessory protein-like (AcPL), is related and similar to IL1RacP and does not bind ligand directly, but rather binds to the complex formed by the IL-18/IL-18Rα chain generating the likely high affinity complex [64]. IL-18β chain is indispensable for activation of NF-kB and c-Jun N-terminal kinase (JNK) in response to IL-18 [65]. Recently, a naturally occurring inhibitor of IL-18, IL-18 binding protein (BP), was described [66, 67]. IL-18BP is secreted in soluble form because it lacks a transmembrane domain. IL-18BP can block binding of mature IL-18 to IL-18R, resulting in the inhibition of IL-18-induced IFN-γ production [66, 67].

Time course studies localizing IL-18 in the pregnant uterus indicate that the entire decidua on gestation day 4 produces IL-18 [68]. IL-18 production starts in the basal proliferative stroma, followed by weaker staining of glandular cells in the normal peri-implantation murine uterus [69]. Transient, very strong labeling of uNK cells by anti-IL-18 antibodies appears in the immediate postimplantation period. IL-18 appears early in murine spongiotrophoblast [69], but not in human villous trophoblast cells [70]. Later on, IL-18 staining persists in giant extravillous trophoblast cells and rare activated macrophages of both species, mice and humans [69, 70] (fig. 1). IL-18 is capable of inducing Fas receptor in amniochorion [71]. There is the possibility that IL-18 by influencing Fas expression on extravillous trophoblast regulates trophoblast invasion (fig. 1).

IL-18R mRNA was detected in epithelial and stromal cells of human endometrial tissue [72]. Also, Tokmadzic et al. [70] demonstrated IL-18R expression on human first trimester villous trophoblast cells. The expression of IL-18BP was demonstrated both in epithelial and stromal cells but there are no findings about its expression in first trimester pregnancy decidua [72]. In view of this data, it is possible that a systemic increase of IL-18 could be involved in the rejection of the maternal-fetal unit through IL-18R, although the presence of IL-18BP in decidual tissue could modify the reaction (fig. 1).

Role of IL-18 on Cytokine Production

The most prominent biological significance of IL-18 is induction of IFN-γ production from Th1 and nonpolarized T cells, NK, B cells and dendritic cells [73–75]. IL-18 by itself induces only a small amount of IFN-γ in anti-CD3-stimulated T cells, but a combination of IL-12 and IL-18 can synergistically induce IFN-γ production [76–78]. Human T cells also require stimulation with both IL-12 and IL-18 to produce significant amounts of IFN-γ [79]. Human CD4+ T cells (CD4+ CD45RA+ T cells) increased their expression of IL-18Rα after being stimulated with IL-12 and displayed dose-dependent IFN-γ production and cell proliferation in response to IL-18 [79, 80]. Contrary to the synergistic effect of IL-18 and IL-12 on the Th1-mediated response, IL-18 itself has the potential to induce IL-4 and IL-13 production in T cells, NK cells, mast cells and basophiles and promotes a Th2-mediated response [81]. Also, IL-18 possesses several biological properties such as regulation of GM-CSF production [82], induction of TNF-α, IL-1β, IL-8, CC and CXC chemokines [83] (fig. 1). IL-18 should be seen as a unique cytokine that enhances innate immunity and both Th1- and Th2-driven immune responses, depending on its cytokine milieu [81]. IL-18 might be of importance in regulating trophoblast invasion and adhesion through its ability to induce production of different chemokines.

IL-12 and IL-18 present at the peri-implantation site could stimulate murine uNK cells to produce IFN-γ that plays key role in vascular remodeling during early pregnancy [84] (N98) (fig. 1). IFN-γ might restrain proinflammatory immune response caused by implantation by enhancing IL-1R antagonist and IL-18BP production that downregulate biological activity of IL-1 or IL-18, respectively [85] (fig. 1). Induction of apoptosis of activated macrophages and particularly T and B cells by IFN-γ [85] might occur in normal early pregnancy decidua and might affect specific distribution of leukocyte cell populations with predominance of NK cells (fig. 1). On the other hand, it has been reported that high levels of IFN-γ and TNF-α are results of an IL-18/IL-12 synergic effect, and thus higher levels of IL-18 in the absence of high IL-12 levels might indeed be beneficial [86].

Role of IL-18 on the Cytolytic Potential

Another important feature of IL-18 is its role in expression of cytotoxic mediators. IL-18- or IL-18Rα-deficient mice have almost the same number of NK cells, but show reduced cytolytic activity against NK cell targets [87]. IL-18 directly upregulates cytotoxic activity of NK cells and CD8+ T cells [76, 88, 89]. IL-18 itself has an extensive ability to induce cell apoptosis by increasing Fas ligand/Fas receptor and granzyme expression on NK, NK/T and CD8+ T cells [81, 89]. It is also known that IL-18 induces perforin expression in NK cells [88]. Moreover, IL-18 upregulates the perforin-dependent cytotoxic activity and FasL-mediated killing of NK cells, but does not enhance their TRAIL expression [89, 90]. Although IL-18 and IL-12 synergistically induce the production of

IFN-γ by NK cells, the two cytokines do not synergize for the upregulation of their cytotoxic activities and it has been shown that IL-18 activates the cytotoxicity of CD8+ T cells independently of IL-12 [91]. This finding may indicate that the activation of the signal transduction system for IFN-γ production is not the same as that for perforin and granzyme-mediated cytotoxicity.

There are only few studies that have investigated IL-18 and its influence on the cytolytic potential of decidual NK cells [69–72]. Tokmadzic et al. [70] have shown that stimulation of DL with IL-18 increases both perforin protein expression and perforin-mediated cytotoxicity against NK-sensitive K562 cells (fig. 1). The combination of IL-12 and IL-18 synergistically increases perforin-mediated activity of early pregnancy peripheral blood lymphocytes by activation of IRAK and NF-kB transcription factor through IL-18 [92] and JAK-STAT signaling pathway through IL-12 [93, 94]. All this acts as a very strong stimulus for perforin exocytosis. Contrary to peripheral blood lymphocytes, IL-12 and IL-18 stimulation of DL significantly increases perforin expression and perforin-mediated cytotoxicity, but does not exceed values obtained by IL-18 stimulation [70]. IL-4, IL-10 and TGF-β, abundantly present in decidua [95], downregulate IL-12R expression [96], possibly ensuring functional inefficiency of IL-12 cytokine. Furthermore, GM-CSF, produced by decidual cells [97], efficiently suppresses IL-12, IL-12-induced IFN-γ production and cytotoxicity of DL in vitro [98].

Since both cytokines, IL-15 and IL-18, are present at the maternal-fetal interface, and they are strong stimulators of cytolytic activity, their effects on cytolytic potential of DL could be important for the control of local cytolytic potential at the interface (fig. 1). Tokmadzic et al. [70] have shown that the combination of IL-15 and IL-18 synergistically enhances the percentage of perforin-positive DL, as well as the average number of perforin protein per cell, but enhanced perforin-mediated cytotoxicity has not been achieved. It is known that IL-15 upregulates inhibitory NK cell receptor, CD94/NKG2A [44], which in turn might inhibit IL-18-mediated cytolytic activity of DL (fig. 1).

Biological Significance of IL-18 at the Maternal-Fetal Interface

IL-18 has an important role in the host defense against intracellular microbes (viruses, bacteria, fungi and protozoa) and against various types of tumors [81]. On the other hand, the excessive production of IL-18 may induce local or systemic injury in the host, as reported for the ontogenesis of autoimmune diseases [81]. Thus, IL-18 could be a double-edged sword that may require tight regulation.

There is a significant elevation of human IL-18 levels in sera from the first trimester until the onset of labor compared to nonpregnant women [99]. Once labor began, IL-18 levels increased further and remained at a high level until at least the third day of puerperium [99]. Elevation of IL-18 in early pregnancy indicates the possible role of IL-18 during implantation. However, there are reports of high levels of IL-18 in sera of women with unexplained implantation failure (NK-IL-18 group) [100], complicated pregnancies (acute fatty liver of pregnancy, fetal growth restriction or preterm premature rupture of membrane) [99] as well as of increased pre-pregnancy serum levels of IL-18 in women with a history of recurrent miscarriage [101, 102]. An increased level of IL-18 promotes strong NK activation and probably excessive IFN-γ production and this state could reflect an inadequate uterine control of NK proliferation and activation (fig. 1). Indeed, the same mechanisms are supposed to be involved in IL-18 and IL-12-induced abortions in mice [103, 104]. On the other hand, implantation sites of IL-18-ablated mice had unmodified spiral arteries [87]. Since it is known that IL-18 is a major enhancer of IL-12-promoted IFN-γ production and IFN-γ is a regulatory cytokine involved in remodeling of decidual arteries [81], this suggests that IL-18 might be necessary for proper vascularization of the implantation site. An IL-18-rich environment would bias the NK cells towards dominance of their activation receptors and induction of cell division and synthesis of IFN-γ and perforin. It seems that the tight regulation of IL-18 expression is important for normal implantation and decidual remodeling events in early pregnancy.

Conclusions

We propose a model (fig. 1) which shows the main aspects of IL-15 and IL-18 action(s) at the maternal-fetal interface and their interplay with various cytokines expressed/produced at this interface.

Acknowledgments

The investigation presented here was financially supported by grants of Croatian Ministry of Science (No. 0062029) and by EC (FVI, Network of Excellence, EMBIC, Contract No. LSHM-CT-2004-512040).

The authors of this manuscript are members of an European Network of Excellence, entitled 'EMBIC' (Embryo Implantation Control), supported by the European Union (contract no. 512040).

References

1 Grabstein KH, Eisenman J, Shanebeck K, Rauch C, Srinivasan S, Fung V, Beers C, Richardson J, Schoenborn MA, Ahdieh M: Cloning of a T cell growth factor that interacts with the beta chain of the interleukin-2 receptor. Science 1994;264:965–968.

2 Bamford RN, Grant AJ, Burton JD, Peters C, Kurys G, Goldman CK, Brennan J, Roessler E, Waldmann TA: The interleukin (IL) 2 receptor beta chain is shared by IL-2 and a cytokine, provisionally designated IL-T, that stimulates T-cell proliferation and the induction of lymphokine-activated killer cells. Proc Natl Acad Sci USA 1994;91:4940–4944.
3 Mrozek E, Anderson P, Caligiuri MA: Role of interleukin-15 in the development of human CD56+ natural killer cells from CD34+ hematopoietic progenitor cells. Blood 1996;87: 2632–2640.
4 Cavazzana-Calvo M, Hacein-Bey S, de Saint Basile G, De Coene C, Selz F, Le Deist F, Fischer A: Role of interleukin-2 (IL-2), IL-7, and IL-15 in natural killer cell differentiation from cord blood hematopoietic progenitor cells and from gamma c transduced severe combined immunodeficiency X1 bone marrow cells. Blood 1996;88:3901–3909.
5 Fraser JD, Irving BA, Crabtree GR, Weiss A: Regulation of interleukin-2 gene enhancer activity by the T cell accessory molecule CD28. Science 1991;251:313–316.
6 Granucci F, Vizzardelli C, Pavelka N, Feau S, Persico M, Virzi E, Rescigno M, Moro G, Ricciardi-Castagnoli P: Inducible IL-2 production by dendritic cells revealed by global gene expression analysis. Nat Immunol 2001;2:882–888.
7 Jokhi PP, King A, Sharkey AM, Smith SK, Loke YW: Screening for cytokine messenger ribonucleic acids in purified human decidual lymphocyte populations by the reverse-transcriptase polymerase chain reaction. J Immunol 1994;153:4427–4435.
8 Giri JG, Ahdieh M, Eisenman J, Shanebeck K, Grabstein K, Kumaki S, Namen A, Park LS, Cosman D, Anderson D: Utilization of the beta and gamma chains of the IL-2 receptor by the novel cytokine IL-15. EMBO J 1994;13:2822–2830.
9 Kennedy MK, Park LS: Characterization of interleukin-15 (IL-15) and the IL-15 receptor complex. J Clin Immunol 1996;16:134–143.
10 Hatakeyama M, Tsudo M, Minamoto S, Kono T, Doi T, Miyata T, Miyasaka M, Taniguchi T: Interleukin-2 receptor beta chain gene: Generation of three receptor forms by cloned human alpha and beta chain cDNA's. Science 1989;244:551–556.
11 Takeshita T, Asao H, Ohtani K, Ishii N, Kumaki S, Tanaka N, Munakata H, Nakamura M, Sugamura K: Cloning of the gamma chain of the human IL-2 receptor. Science 1992;257: 379–382.
12 Nishikawa K, Saito S, Morii T, Hamada K, Ako H, Narita N, Ichijo M, Kurahayashi M, Sugamura K: Accumulation of CD16–CD56+ natural killer cells with high affinity interleukin 2 receptors in human early pregnancy decidua. Int Immunol 1991;3:743–750.
13 King A, Wheeler R, Carter NP, Francis DP, Loke YW: The response of human decidual leukocytes to IL-2. Cell Immunol 1992;141:409–421.
14 Starkey PM: Expression on cells of early human pregnancy decidua, of the p75, IL-2 and p145, IL-4 receptor proteins. Immunology 1991;73:64–70.
15 Verma S, Hiby SE, Loke YW, King A: Human decidual natural killer cells express the receptor for and respond to the cytokine interleukin 15. Biol Reprod 2000;62:959–968.
16 Giri JG, Anderson DM, Kumaki S, Park LS, Grabstein KH, Cosman D: IL-15, a novel T cell growth factor that shares activities and receptor components with IL-2. J Leukoc Biol 1995; 57:763–766.
17 Anderson DM, Kumaki S, Ahdieh M, Bertles J, Tometsko M, Loomis A, Giri J, Copeland NG, Gilbert DJ, Jenkins NA: Functional characterization of the human interleukin-15 receptor alpha chain and close linkage of IL15RA and IL2RA genes. J Biol Chem 1995;270:29862–29869.
18 Ye W, Zheng LM, Young JD, Liu CC: The involvement of interleukin (IL)-15 in regulating the differentiation of granulated metrial gland cells in mouse pregnant uterus. J Exp Med 1996;184: 2405–2410.
19 Okada S, Okada H, Sanezumi M, Nakajima T, Yasuda K, Kanzaki H: Expression of interleukin-15 in human endometrium and decidua. Mol Hum Reprod 2000;6:75–80.
20 Kitaya K, Yasuda J, Yagi I, Tada Y, Fushiki S, Honjo H: IL-15 expression at human endometrium and decidua. Biol Reprod 2000;63:683–687.
21 Fortunato SJ, Menon R, Lombardi SJ: IL-15, a novel cytokine produced by human fetal membranes, is elevated in preterm labor. Am J Reprod Immunol 1998;39:16–23.

22 Okada H, Nakajima T, Sanezumi M, Ikuta A, Yasuda K, Kanzaki H: Progesterone enhances interleukin-15 production in human endometrial stromal cells in vitro. J Clin Endocrinol Metab 2000;85:4765–4770.
23 Loke YW, King A, Burrows TD: Decidua in human implantation. Hum Reprod 1995;10:14–21.
24 Kao LC, Germeyer A, Tulac S, Lobo S, Yang JP, Taylor RN, Osteen K, Lessey BA, Giudice LC: Expression profiling of endometrium from women with endometriosis reveals candidate genes for disease-based implantation failure and infertility. Endocrinology 2003;144:2870–2881.
25 Chegini N, Ma C, Roberts M, Williams RS, Ripps BA: Differential expression of interleukins (IL) IL-13 and IL-15 throughout the menstrual cycle in endometrium of normal fertile women and women with recurrent spontaneous abortion. J Reprod Immunol 2002;56:93–110.
26 Okada H, Nakajima T, Yasuda K, Kanzaki H: Interleukin-1 inhibits interleukin-15 production by progesterone during in vitro decidualization in human. J Reprod Immunol 2004;61:3–12.
27 Khan IA, Kasper LH: IL-15 augments CD8+ T cell-mediated immunity against *Toxoplasma gondii* infection in mice. J Immunol 1996;157:2103–2108.
28 Xin KQ, Hamajima K, Sasaki S, Tsuji T, Watabe S, Okada E, Okuda K: IL-15 expression plasmid enhances cell-mediated immunity induced by an HIV-1 DNA vaccine. Vaccine 1999;17:858–866.
29 Masuda A, Matsuguchi T, Yamaki K, Hayakawa T, Kubo M, LaRochelle WJ, Yoshikai Y: Interleukin-15 induces rapid tyrosine phosphorylation of STAT6 and the expression of interleukin-4 in mouse mast cells. J Biol Chem 2000;275:29331–29337.
30 Mori A, Suko M, Kaminuma O, Inoue S, Ohmura T, Nishizaki Y, Nagahori T, Asakura Y, Hoshino A, Okumura Y, Sato G, Ito K, Okudaira H: IL-15 promotes cytokine production of human T helper cells. J Immunol 1996;156:2400–2405.
31 Ruckert R, Herz U, Paus R, Ungureanu D, Pohl T, Renz H, Bulfone-Paus S: IL-15-IgG2b fusion protein accelerates and enhances a Th2 but not a Th1 immune response in vivo, while IL-2-IgG2b fusion protein inhibits both. Eur J Immunol 1998;28:3312–3320.
32 Carson WE, Giri JG, Lindemann MJ, Linett ML, Ahdieh M, Paxton R, Anderson D, Eisenmann J, Grabstein K, Caligiuri MA: Interleukin (IL) 15 is a novel cytokine that activates human natural killer cells via components of the IL-2 receptor. J Exp Med 1994;180:1395–1403.
33 Fehniger TA, Carson WE, Caligiuri MA: Costimulation of human natural killer cells is required for interferon gamma production. Transplant Proc 1999;31:1476–1478.
34 Fehniger TA, Shah MH, Turner MJ, VanDeusen JB, Whitman SP, Cooper MA, Suzuki K, Wechser M, Goodsaid F, Caligiuri MA: Differential cytokine and chemokine gene expression by human NK cells following activation with IL-18 or IL-15 in combination with IL-12: Implications for the innate immune response. J Immunol 1999;162:4511–4520.
35 Bluman EM, Bartynski KJ, Avalos BR, Caligiuri MA: Human natural killer cells produce abundant macrophage inflammatory protein-1 alpha in response to monocyte-derived cytokines. J Clin Invest 1996;97:2722–2727.
36 Maghazachi AA, al-Aoukaty A, Schall TJ: C-C chemokines induce the chemotaxis of NK and IL-2-activated NK cells. Role for G proteins. J Immunol 1994;153:4969–4977.
37 Fahey TJ 3rd, Tracey KJ, Tekamp-Olson P, Cousens LS, Jones WG, Shires GT, Cerami A, Sherry B: Macrophage inflammatory protein 1 modulates macrophage function. J Immunol 1992;148: 2764–2769.
38 Cooper MA, Fehniger TA, Turner SC, Chen KS, Ghaheri BA, Ghayur T, Carson WE, Caligiuri MA: Human natural killer cells: A unique innate immunoregulatory role for the CD56(bright) subset. Blood 2001;97:3146–3151.
39 Eriksson M, Meadows SK, Wira CR, Sentman CL: Unique phenotype of human uterine NK cells and their regulation by endogenous TGF-beta. J Leukoc Biol 2004;76:667–675.
40 Atedzoe BN, Ahmad A, Menezes J: Enhancement of natural killer cell cytotoxicity by the human herpesvirus-7 via IL-15 induction. J Immunol 1997;159:4966–4972.
41 Rukavina D, Bogovic T, Sotosek V, Laskarin G, Strbo N, Juretic K, Cupurdija K, Tsuji Y, Koyama K: Physiological role(s) of IL-15 and IL-18 at the maternal-fetal (m-f) interface. 8th Congress of the AASIR, Weimar, Germany. Am J Reprod Immunol 2002;48:139.
42 Vitale M, Bottino C, Sivori S, Sanseverino L, Castriconi R, Marcenaro E, Augugliaro R, Moretta L, Moretta A: NKp44, a novel triggering surface molecule specifically expressed by activated natural

killer cells, is involved in non-major histocompatibility complex-restricted tumor cell lysis. J Exp Med 1998;187:2065–2072.
43 Sivori S, Pende D, Bottino C, Marcenaro E, Pessino A, Biassoni R, Moretta L, Moretta A: NKp46 is the major triggering receptor involved in the natural cytotoxicity of fresh or cultured human NK cells. Correlation between surface density of NKp46 and natural cytotoxicity against autologous, allogeneic or xenogeneic target cells. Eur J Immunol 1999;29:1656–1666.
44 Mingari MC, Vitale C, Cantoni C, Bellomo R, Ponte M, Schiavetti F, Bertone S, Moretta A, Moretta L: Interleukin-15-induced maturation of human natural killer cells from early thymic precursors: Selective expression of CD94/NKG2-A as the only HLA class I-specific inhibitory receptor. Eur J Immunol 1997;27:1374–1380.
45 Strbo N, Laskarin G, Sotosek V, Randic LJ, Rukavina D: Regulation of cytolytic activity of decidual lymphocytes: Role of cytokines IL-2 and IL-15. IFPA Meeting 1999, 8th Meeting of the European Placenta Group, Schladming, Austria. Placenta 1999;20:A64.
46 Bogovic Crncic T, Strbo N, Laskarin G, Cupurdija K, Dorcic D, Juretic K, Dupor J, Sotosek Tokmadzic V, Vlastelic I, Randic LJ, Rukavina D: Decidual NK cells use Fas/FasL cytolytic pathway, European Congress of Reproductive Immunology, Pilsen, Czech Republic. Am J Reprod Immunol 2004;51:490.
47 Strbo N, Laskarin G, Sotosek V, Randic LJ, Podack ER, Rukavina D: Modulation of perforin expression in the decidual and peripheral blood cytotoxic lymphocytes in culture. Am J Reprod Immunol 1999;42:14–21.
48 Sotosek V, Laskarin G, Strbo N, Dohr G, Blaschitz A, Podack ER, Rukavina D: Decidual macrophages are the population of decidual adherent cells which regulates perforin expression in cytolytic cells. Am J Reprod Immunol 1999;42:76–82.
49 Rukavina D, Podack ER: Abundant perforin expression at the maternal-fetal interface: Guarding the semiallogeneic transplant? Immunol Today 2000;21:160–163.
50 Kauma S, Huff T, Krystal G, Ryan J, Takacs P, Turner T: The expression of stem cell factor and its receptor, c-kit in human endometrium and placental tissues during pregnancy. J Clin Endocrinol Metab 1996;81:1261–1266.
51 Carson WE, Fehniger TA, Caligiuri MA: CD56bright natural killer cell subsets: Characterization of distinct functional responses to interleukin-2 and the c-kit ligand. Eur J Immunol 1997; 27:354–360.
52 Umekage H, Saito S, Morikawa H: Enhancement by stem cell factor of interleukin-2 (IL-2)-induced DNA synthesis in human decidual CD16– CD56bright natural killer cells mediated by increased expression of the IL-2 receptor alpha chain. J Reprod Immunol 1998;40:1–24.
53 Carayol G, Robin C, Bourhis JH, Bennaceur-Griscelli A, Chouaib S, Coulombel L, Caignard A: NK cells differentiated from bone marrow, cord blood and peripheral blood stem cells exhibit similar phenotype and functions. Eur J Immunol 1998;28:1991–2002.
54 Ashkar AA, Black GP, Wei Q, He H, Liang L, Head JR, Croy BA: Assessment of requirements for IL-15 and IFN regulatory factors in uterine NK cell differentiation and function during pregnancy. J Immunol 2003;171:2937–2944.
55 Lodolce JP, Boone DL, Chai S, Swain RE, Dassopoulos T, Trettin S, Ma A: IL-15 receptor maintains lymphoid homeostasis by supporting lymphocyte homing and proliferation. Immunity 1998; 9:669–676.
56 Carson WE, Haldar S, Baiocchi RA, Croce CM, Caligiuri MA: The c-kit ligand suppresses apoptosis of human natural killer cells through the upregulation of bcl-2. Proc Natl Acad Sci USA 1994;91:7553–7557.
57 Bulfone-Paus S, Ungureanu D, Pohl T, Lindner G, Paus R, Ruckert R, Krause H, Kunzendorf U: Interleukin-15 protects from lethal apoptosis in vivo. Nat Med 1997;3:1124–1128.
58 Alleva DG, Kaser SB, Monroy MA, Fenton MJ, Beller DI: IL-15 functions as a potent autocrine regulator of macrophage proinflammatory cytokine production: Evidence for differential receptor subunit utilization associated with stimulation or inhibition. J Immunol 1997;159:2941–2951.
59 Ghayur T, Banerjee S, Hugunin M, Butler D, Herzog L, Carter A, Quintal L, Sekut L, Talanian R, Paskind M, Wong W, Kamen R, Tracey D, Allen H: Caspase-1 processes IFN-gamma-inducing factor and regulates LPS-induced IFN-gamma production. Nature 1997;386:619–623.

60 McInnes IB, Gracie JA, Leung BP, Wei XQ, Liew FY: Interleukin 18: A pleiotropic participant in chronic inflammation. Immunol Today 2000;21:312–315.
61 Torigoe K, Ushio S, Okura T, Kobayashi S, Taniai M, Kunikata T, Murakami T, Sanou O, Kojima H, Fujii M, Ohta T, Ikeda M, Ikegami H, Kurimoto M: Purification and characterization of the human interleukin-18 receptor. J Biol Chem 1997;272:25737–25742.
62 Parnet P, Garka KE, Bonnert TP, Dower SK, Sims JE: IL-1Rrp is a novel receptor-like molecule similar to the type I interleukin-1 receptor and its homologues T1/ST2 and IL-1R AcP. J Biol Chem 1996;271:3967–3970.
63 Kanakaraj P, Ngo K, Wu Y, Angulo A, Ghazal P, Harris CA, Siekierka JJ, Peterson PA, Fung-Leung WP: Defective interleukin (IL)-18-mediated natural killer and T helper cell type 1 responses in IL-1 receptor-associated kinase (IRAK)-deficient mice. J Exp Med 1999;189: 1129–1138.
64 Dinarello CA: Interleukin-18. Methods 1999;19:121–132.
65 Reznikov LL, Kim SH, Zhou L, Bufler P, Goncharov I, Tsang M, Dinarello CA: The combination of soluble IL-18Ralpha and IL-18Rbeta chains inhibits IL-18-induced IFN-gamma. J Interferon Cytokine Res 2002;22:593–601.
66 Novick D, Kim SH, Fantuzzi G, Reznikov LL, Dinarello CA, Rubinstein M: Interleukin-18 binding protein: A novel modulator of the Th1 cytokine response. Immunity 1999;10:127–136.
67 Kim S-H, Eisenstein M, Reznikov L: Structural requirements of six naturally occurring isoforms of the IL-18 binding protein to inhibit IL-18. Proc Natl Acad Sci USA 2000;97:1190–1195.
68 Chaouat G, Zourbas S, Ostojic S, Lappree-Delage G, Dubanchet S, Ledee N, Martal J: A brief review of recent data on some cytokine expressions at the materno-foetal interface which might challenge the classical Th1/Th2 dichotomy. J Reprod Immunol 2002;53:241–256.
69 Ostojic S, Dubanchet S, Chaouat G, Abdelkarim M, Truyens C, Capron F: Demonstration of the presence of IL-16, IL-17 and IL-18 at the murine fetomaternal interface during murine pregnancy. Am J Reprod Immunol 2003;49:101–112.
70 Tokmadzic VS, Tsuji Y, Bogovic T, Laskarin G, Cupurdija K, Strbo N, Koyama K, Okamura H, Podack ER, Rukavina D: IL-18 is present at the maternal-fetal interface and enhances cytotoxic activity of decidual lymphocytes. Am J Reprod Immunol 2002;48:191–200.
71 Menon R, Lombardi SJ, Fortunato SJ: IL-18, a product of choriodecidual cells, increases during premature rupture of membranes but fails to turn on the Fas-FasL-mediated apoptosis pathway. J Assist Reprod Genet 2001;18:276–284.
72 Yoshino O, Osuga Y, Koga K, Tsutsumi O, Yano T, Fujii T, Kugu K, Momoeda M, Fujiwara T, Tomita K, Taketani Y: Evidence for the expression of interleukin (IL)-18, IL-18 receptor and IL-18 binding protein in the human endometrium. Mol Hum Reprod 2001;7:649–654.
73 Nakamura K, Okamura H, Wada M, Nagata K, Tamura T: Endotoxin-induced serum factor that stimulates gamma interferon production. Infect Immun 1989;57:590–595.
74 Cai G, Kastelein RA, Hunter CA: IL-10 enhances NK cell proliferation, cytotoxicity and production of IFN-gamma when combined with IL-18. Eur J Immunol 1999;29:2658–2665.
75 Yoshimoto T, Okamura H, Tagawa YI, Iwakura Y, Nakanishi K: Interleukin 18 together with interleukin 12 inhibits IgE production by induction of interferon-gamma production from activated B cells. Proc Natl Acad Sci USA 1997;94:3948–3953.
76 Okamura H, Tsutsui H, Komatsu T: Cloning of a new cytokine that induces IFN-gamma production by T cells. Nature 1995;378:88–91.
77 Yoshimoto T, Takeda K, Tanaka T: IL-12 up-regulates IL-18 receptor expression on T cells, Th1 cells, and B cells: Synergism with IL-18 for IFN-gamma production. J Immunol 1998;161:3400–3407.
78 Micallef MJ, Ohtsuki T, Kohno K: Interferon-γ-inducing factor enhances T helper 1 cytokine production by stimulated human T cells: Synergism with interleukin-12 for interferon-gamma production. Eur J Immunol 1996;26:1647–1651.
79 Tominaga K, Yoshimoto T, Torigoe K: IL-12 synergizes with IL-18 or IL-1b for IFN-gamma production from human T cells. Int Immunol 2000;12:151–160.
80 Kunikata T, Torigoe K, Ushio S: Constitutive and induced IL-18 receptor expression by various peripheral blood cell subsets as determined by anti-hIL-18R monoclonal antibody. Cell Immunol 1998;189:135–143.

81 Nakanishi K, Yoshimoto T, Tsutsui H, Okamura H: Interleukin-18 is a unique cytokine that stimulates both Th1 and Th2 responses depending on its cytokine milieu. Cytokine Growth Factor Rev 2001;12:53–72.
82 Robertson SA, O'Connell AC, Hudson SN, Seamark RF: Granulocyte-macrophage colony-stimulating factor (GM-CSF) targets myeloid leukocytes in the uterus during the post-mating inflammatory response in mice. J Reprod Immunol 2000;46:131–154.
83 Puren AJ, Fantuzzi G, Gu Y, Su MS, Dinarello CA: Interleukin-18 (IFNgamma-inducing factor) induces IL-8 and IL-1beta via TNFalpha production from non-CD14+ human blood mononuclear cells. J Clin Invest 1998;101:711–721.
84 Croy BA, Esadeg S, Chantakru S, van den Heuvel M, Paffaro VA, He H, Black GP, Ashkar AA, Kiso Y, Zhang J: Update on pathways regulating the activation of uterine natural killer cells, their interactions with decidual spiral arteries and homing of their precursors to the uterus. J Reprod Immunol 2003;59:175–191
85 Muhl H, Pfeilschifter J: Anti-inflammatory properties of pro-inflammatory interferon-gamma. Int Immunopharmacol 2003;3:1247–1255.
86 Dinarello CA, Novick D, Puren AJ, Fantuzzi G, Shapiro L, Muhl H, Yoon DY, Reznikov LL, Kim SH, Rubinstein M: Overview of interleukin-18: More than an interferon-gamma inducing factor. J Leukoc Biol 1998;63:658–664.
87 Takeda K, Tsutsui H, Yoshimoto T, Adachi O, Yoshida N, Kishimoto T, Okamura H, Nakanishi K, Akira S: Defective NK cell activity and Th1 response in IL-18-deficient mice. Immunity 1998; 8:383–390.
88 Hyodo Y, Matsui K, Hayashi N: IL-18 up-regulates perforin-mediated NK activity without increasing perforin messenger RNA expression by binding to constitutively expressed IL-18 receptor. J Immunol 1999;162:1662–1668.
89 Tsutsui H, Nakanishi K, Matsui K: Interferon-γ-inducing factor up-regulates Fas ligand-mediated cytotoxic activity of murine natural killer cell clones. J Immunol 1996;157:3967–3973.
90 Kayagaki N, Yamaguchi N, Nakayama M, et al: Expression and function of TNF-related apoptosis-inducing ligand (TRAIL) on murine activated NK cells. J Immunol 1999;163:1906–1913.
91 Kohyama M, Saijyo K, Hayasida M, Yasugi T, Kurimoto M, Ohno T: Direct activation of human CD8+ cytotoxic T lymphocytes by interleukin-18. Jpn J Cancer Res 1998;89:1016–1041.
92 Robinson D, Shibuya K, Mui A, Zonin F, Murphy E, Sana T, Hartley SB, Menon S, Kastelein R, Bazan F, O'Garra A: IGIF does not drive Th1 development but synergizes with IL-12 for interferon-gamma production and activates IRAK and NFkappaB. Immunity 1997;7:571–581.
93 Bacon CM, Petricoin EF 3rd, Ortaldo JR, Rees RC, Larner AC, Johnston JA, O'Shea JJ: Interleukin 12 induces tyrosine phosphorylation and activation of STAT4 in human lymphocytes. Proc Natl Acad Sci USA 1995;92:7307–7311.
94 Bacon CM, McVicar DW, Ortaldo JR, Rees RC, O'Shea JJ, Johnston JA: Interleukin 12 (IL-12) induces tyrosine phosphorylation of JAK2 and TYK2: Differential use of Janus family tyrosine kinases by IL-2 and IL-12. J Exp Med 1995;181:399–404.
95 Chaouat G, Cayol V, Mairovitz V, Dubanchet S: Localization of the Th2 cytokines IL-3, IL-4, IL-10 at the fetomaternal interface during human and murine pregnancy and lack of requirement for Fas/Fas ligand interaction for a successful allogeneic pregnancy. Am J Reprod Immunol 1999; 42:1–13.
96 Wu C, Warrier RR, Wang X, Presky DH, Gately MK: Regulation of interleukin-12 receptor beta1 chain expression and interleukin-12 binding by human peripheral blood mononuclear cells. Eur J Immunol 1997;27:147–154.
97 Miyama M, Umesaki N, Kawabata M: Identification of the granulocyte colony-stimulating factor (G-CSF) producing cell population in human decidua and its biological action on trophoblast cell. Osaka City Med J 1998;44:85–96.
98 Sugita K, Hayakawa S, Karasaki-Suzuki M, Hagiwara H, Chishima F, Aleemuzaman S, Li JA, Nishinarita S, Yamamoto T: Granulocyte colony stimulation factor (G-CSF) suppresses interleukin (IL)-12 and/or IL-2 induced interferon (IFN)-gamma production and cytotoxicity of decidual mononuclear cells. Am J Reprod Immunol 2003;50:83–89.

99 Ida A, Tsuji Y, Muranaka J, Kanazawa R, Nakata Y, Adachi S, Okamura H, Koyama K: IL-18 in pregnancy; the elevation of IL-18 in maternal peripheral blood during labour and complicated pregnancies. J Reprod Immunol 2000;47:65–74.
100 Ledee-Bataille N, Dubanchet S, Coulomb-L'Hermine A, Durand-Gasselin I, Frydman R, Chaouat G: A new role for natural killer cells, interleukin (IL)-12, and IL-18 in repeated implantation failure after in vitro fertilization. Fertil Steril 2004;81:59–65.
101 Jacobsson B, Holst RM, Mattsby-Baltzer I, Nikolaitchouk N, Wennerholm UB, Hagberg H: Interleukin-18 in cervical mucus and amniotic fluid: Relationship to microbial invasion of the amniotic fluid, intra-amniotic inflammation and preterm delivery. BJOG 2003;110:598–603.
102 Wilson R, Jenkins C, Miller H, McInnes IB, Moore J, McLean MA, Walker JJ: Abnormal cytokine levels in non-pregnant women with a history of recurrent miscarriage. Eur J Obstet Gynecol Reprod Biol 2004;115:51–54.
103 Clark DA, Chaouat G, Arck PC, Mittruecker HW, Levy GA: Cytokine-dependent abortion in CBA × DBA/2 mice is mediated by the procoagulant fgl2 prothrombinase (correction of prothombinase). J Immunol 1998;160:545–549.
104 Zenclussen AC, Joachim R, Hagen E, Peiser C, Klapp BF, Arck PC: Heme oxygenase is downregulated in stress-triggered and interleukin-12-mediated murine abortion. Scand J Immunol 2002; 55:560–569.

Daniel Rukavina
Department of Physiology and Immunology
Medical Faculty, University of Rijeka, Brace Branchetta 20
HR–Rijeka 51 000 (Croatia), Tel. +385 51 65 11 50
Fax +385 51 67 56 99, E-Mail daniel@medri.hr

Markert UR (ed): Immunology of Pregnancy.
Chem Immunol Allergy. Basel, Karger, 2005, vol 89, pp 26–35

The Possible Role of the JAK/STAT Pathway in Lymphocytes at the Fetomaternal Interface

Tobias G. Poehlmann, Susann Busch, Bianka Mussil, Harald Winzer, Judith Weinert, Imke Mebes, Andreas Schaumann, Justine S. Fitzgerald, Udo R. Markert

Department of Obstetrics, Friedrich Schiller University, Jena, Germany

Abstract

Pregnancy is accompanied by a Th2-prone immune modulation, which is a major puzzle piece among maternofetal tolerance-promoting factors. A large number of cytokines is physiologically or pathologically present in the decidua and is potentially able to act on lymphocytes and NK cells, which express a variety of respective receptors. Intracellular signals from these receptors are to a major part transduced via the Janus kinases (JAK) and signal transducers and activators of a transcription (STAT) system, which consists of at least 4 different kinases and 7 STATs plus several subtypes and splicing variants. A network of suppressors of cytokine signaling (SOCS) controls their balance. The interactions of all these intracellular factors and cross-linking with further signaling systems seem to be crucial for the maintenance of a maternal cytokine profile which promotes the tolerance of the fetus.

Introduction

Lymphocytes at the Fetomaternal Interface

During the menstrual cycle, the number of CD45+ leukocytes increases premenstrually from 10–15 to 20–25% of all endometrial cells [1, 2]. During the first trimenon of pregnancy, the number increases further and approximately 70% of immunocompetent decidual cells are CD45+ leukocytes. The predominant type of these cells are transient, pregnancy-associated uterine natural killer cells (46%), followed by macrophages (19%) and T cells (8%), mainly CD8+ T cells [3].

As shown in various knockout animal models, most classes of immune cells are indispensable for successful pregnancy, but their function and way of action are modified compared with leukocytes from peripheral blood, other tissues or inflammation areas. It may be suggested that such modifications are regulated on the signal transduction level.

The JAK/STAT Pathway

Cytokines bind lymphocytes via cytokine receptors, which induces phosphorylation of their intracellular tail through tyrosine kinases. Janus kinases (JAK) represent a major group of them. The phosphorylated receptor tails offer docking sites for SH2-containing signaling proteins which can be phosphorylated at various tyrosine and serine binding sites following their association with the complex [4]. Signal transducers and activators of transcription (STAT) form a major family of substrates of phosphorylation. Phosphorylation at different binding sites of the STATs fundamentally changes function, DNA binding and transcription and is influenced by various further signaling systems such as mitogen-activated protein kinases MAPK/ERK, phosphatidylinositol 3-kinase and calcium/calmodulin-dependent kinase (CaMKII) [5–8] (for details, see Fitzgerald et al., volume 89). Phosphorylated STATs may then form homo- and heterodimers and translocate into the nucleus. After DNA binding, STATs can modulate the expression of target genes [9] and induce negative feedback loops [10]. Positive loops also exist: For example, interleukin-2 (IL-2) induces transcription and production of IL-2 receptor via the JAK-STAT pathway in lymphocytes [11, 12].

Most cytokines use more than one of at least four JAK and seven STAT family members, but also each JAK and STAT molecule is used by several distinct cytokines [4].

Cytokines and Growth Factors in the Decidua with Capacity to Use the JAK/STAT Pathway

A wide spectrum of cytokines and growth factors is present in the decidua physiologically, but can be present pathologically and, thus, signal via the JAK/STAT system. These cytokines include leukemia inhibitory factor, tumor necrosis factor-α, interferon-γ (IFN-γ), IL-1, IL-2, IL-4, IL-5, IL-6, IL-8, IL-10, IL-11, IL-12, IL-13, IL-15, IL-16, and IL-18 [13–16]. These signals may again lead to production and release of a variety of further cytokines. Compared to the general balance of cytokine profiles in the uterus, anti-inflammatory T helper 2

(Th2)-type cytokines are predominant during pregnancy and especially in the decidua [17, 18]. Nonetheless, proinflammatory Th1-type cytokines are present in relatively low concentrations. The potential exists to produce and release these cytokines in response to various stimuli, such as infectious reagents, cell stress, neural transmitters and other factors. It may be expected that the fine-tuned cytokine balance between Th1 and Th2, which is crucial for maintenance of pregnancy, is regulated on the intracellular signaling level, which on the other hand is regulated by cytokines and other factors, thus forming a complex network of intra- and extracellular regulation mechanisms. This includes, to a substantial part, the JAK/STAT system [19]. The availability and susceptibility of these signaling molecules to stimuli may be the key regulator of leukocyte functions in the decidua.

In the following, those mechanisms and factors will be presented and discussed which favor the predominance of Th2 and the downregulation of Th1 cytokines or other potentially dangerous factors for pregnancy.

Signaling in T Cells

Many factors, including the cytokines mentioned, influence and regulate T cell functions. IL-12, IL-2, IL-23 and IL-27 play a major role in the differentiation of naive T cells to that of the Th1 subset, while IL-4 does for differentiation into the Th2 subset [20]. Very little is known about specific intracellular signals in decidual or other lymphocytes during pregnancy that may support maternofetal tolerance. Thus, here we can provide only a brief overview of known JAK/STAT aspects, independent of pregnancy, but which might be involved in the regulation of lymphocytes in pregnancy.

IL-4-Induced Signaling

IL-4 is the essential anti-inflammatory cytokine for Th2 differentiation. It derives from dendritic cells, T cells themselves, mast cells and others. IL-4 is continuously present at the maternal-fetal interface, where it is involved in pregnancy-supporting mechanisms [16, 21, 22]. Progesterone-induced blocking factor is a major inducer of IL-4 production in pregnancy [23, 24]. The IL-4 receptor is a heterodimer. One chain, the IL-4R α-chain, binds IL-4 with high affinity and determines the nature of the biochemical signals that are induced. Although the γ-chain is shared with other inflammatory cytokines, such as IL-2, IL-6, IL-12, IL-15, IL-21 and others, the signaling pathway is different [25]. IL-4 upregulates the transcription of GATA3 via STAT6, which leads to Th2 cytokine production and to a silencing of the IFN-γ production [20, 26]. Mice lacking STAT6 exclusively develop a Th1 response [27].

Furthermore, IL-18 has been well characterized as a costimulatory factor for the induction of IL-12-mediated IFN-γ production by Th1 cells, but it can also induce IL-4 production and thus facilitate the differentiation of Th2 cells. The positive/negative regulation of the IL-18 receptor (IL-18R) α by the major inductive cytokines (IL-12 and IL-4) determines the capacity of IL-18 to polarize an immune response [28].

IL-13-Induced Signaling

IL-13, a cytokine similar to IL-4, is a regulator of human B cell and monocyte functions. Furthermore, IL-13, like IL-4, induces distinct STAT6-DNA binding complexes and tyrosine phosphorylation of STAT6 and Janus kinase 3 (JAK3) in NK and T cells [29].

IL-10-Family-Induced Signaling

IL-10 is a crucial interleukin for the survival of the fetal allograft, which counteracts the effects of deleterious inflammatory cytokines [30]. Binding of cytokines of the IL-10 family to its receptors leads to STAT1 and STAT3 phosporylation via JAK1 [31, 32]. STAT3 seems to be the main, but not unique mediator of IL-10 anti-inflammatory functions [33]. The role of several further cytokines of this group during pregnancy, such as IL-19, IL-20, IL-22, IL-24 and IL-26, is not yet known, although they share the IL-10R, IL-20R and IL-22R and the same intracellular pathways [34].

IL-12-Induced Signaling

IL-12 is produced by antigen-presenting cells, dendritic cells as well as macrophages, and induces Th1-type T cells [35, 36]. It signals through JAK2, Tyk2, STAT3 and STAT4 intracellularly [37]. IL-12 or STAT4-deficient mice are defective in Th1 reactions [38, 39]. High levels of IL-12 during pregnancy are associated with severe disorders, such as preterm labor, preterm birth or recurrent miscarriage [22, 40].

IL-2-Induced Signaling

IL-2 is produced by Th1 cells themselves and is able to initiate an autocrine signal via IL-2 receptors on their own cell surfaces. This leads to a further increase of IL-2 production and release via STAT1, STAT3, STAT5a and STAT5b activation [26, 41, 42]. Simultaneously, MAPKinase and phosphatidylinositol 3-kinase pathways are also activated. Similar receptors and pathways are used by the other IL-2 family cytokines IL-6, IL-12, IL-15 or IL-21 [26, 43]. Incubation of lymphocytes with supernatants from Jeg-3 choriocarcinoma cells reduces the expression of the STAT molecules mentioned, as well as of JAK1 and JAK3, along with cellular activity [41, 44]. Supernatants from trophoblast cells, but also from tumors display similar capacities [45, 46].

IFN-α/β- and IFN-γ-Induced Signaling

IFN-α/β is produced by virally infected cells and plays an important role in early phases of the innate immune response. IFN-α/β inhibits IL-4 signaling in B cells and monocytes, suggesting that IFN-α/β (like IFN-γ) is a Th1 cytokine [47]. IFN-α, IFN-β and, less intensively, IFN-γ are present in the placenta, mostly localized in extravillous interstitial trophoblast, but also in villous syncytiotrophoblast [48]. IFN-α/β induces STAT1, STAT2, STAT3 and STAT4 tyrosine phosphorylation and DNA binding leading to IL-21 expression and downregulation of IL-21R in T cells [49, 50]. IFN-α enhances IL-4-mediated STAT6 activation in CD4+ and CD8+ human T cells. The effect is specific because IFN-γ does not enhance IL-4-mediated STAT6 activation. IFN-α-mediated STAT1 and STAT2 activation is not modulated by IL-4, and activation of Janus kinases is not enhanced or prolonged by simultaneous stimulation with IFN-α and IL-4 [47]. IFN-γ signals mainly via tyrosine phosphorylation of STAT1 and STAT3 [49]. The above-described suppression of JAK/STAT factors by trophoblast or tumor-derived culture supernatants may also reduce potentially harming effects of IFN-γ in pregnancy [40].

Suppressors of Cytokine Signaling

Suppressor of cytokine signaling (SOCS) proteins have emerged as important regulators of cytokine signals in lymphocytes and are constitutively expressed in naive Th cells, albeit at low levels. They are differentially induced by Th-polarizing cytokines. STAT1 signals play major roles in inducing SOCS expression in T helper cells. Induction of SOCS expression by IL-4, IL-12, or IFN-γ is compromised in STAT1-deficient primary Th cells. IL-4 is a potent inducer of STAT1 activation in Th2, but not Th1 cells, and SOCS1 or SOCS3 expression is dramatically reduced in STAT1(–/–) Th2 cells [51]. Overexpression of SOCS1 in Th2 cells represses STAT6 activation and profoundly inhibits IL-4-induced proliferation, while depletion of SOCS1 by an antisense SOCS1 cDNA construct enhances cell proliferation and induces constitutive activation of STAT6 in Th2 cells [51]. In addition to the polarized activation of STAT4 in Th1 cells and STAT6 in Th2 cells, STAT3 and STAT5 are selectively activated in Th1 cells following differentiation that was associated with the differential induction of SOCS molecules. In this way, it could be suggested that STAT3 and STAT5, possibly regulated by the SOCS proteins, may play a role in the differentiation of Th cells, in the maintenance of the Th1 and Th2 phenotype, and, thus, the regulation of the Th1/Th2 cytokine balance [52]. This is supported by the observation that SOCS3 is expressed at high concentrations in Th2 cells, where it inhibits IL-12-induced STAT4 signaling [53].

SOCS1 deficiency in mice leads to lymphocyte-dependent multiorgan disease and perinatal death. Experiments with SOCS1 knockout mice published by Fujimoto et al. [54] suggest that SOCS1 plays a regulatory role in both T(h)1 and T(h)2 polarizations.

SOCS are detected in gestational tissues and their differential regulation is associated with the onset of labor, but no information about their role in decidual or peripheral lymphocytes in pregnancy has been published thus far [55, 56].

JAK/STAT Signaling in NK Cells

To date, little is known about JAK/STAT signal transduction in decidual NK cells. CD56+ NK cells from endometrial tissue express prolactin (PRL) receptor and might be a potential target of the hormone PRL, whose secretion is increased during early pregnancy and decreases to term. PRL engagement triggers tyrosine phosphorylation of JAK2 and STAT1 and STAT5. PRL, like other class I cytokines, also stimulates MAPK/ERK pathway [57]. SOCS1 can prevent intracellular PRL signaling and gene expression in decidual cells [58]. PRL stimulation of NK cells increases expression of IL-2R and IL-15R, perforin and Fas ligand, all events which are potentially harming the fetal allograft, similar to the induction of antitumor cytotoxicity of NK cells through PRL [59, 60]. When female alymphoid recombinase activating gene (RAG)-2 and common cytokine receptor chain-γ knockout mice were grafted with bone marrow from STAT1 knockout donors, uterine NK cells were overexpressed and immature [61].

Optimal NK cell development and activation, as well as cytolytic activity, involves IL-2R β signals that also upregulate expression of the pore-forming effector molecule perforin. IL-2 ligation of its receptor stimulates STAT1, STAT3 and STAT5 [61, 62]. In some NK cell lines it also triggers activation of STAT4 and increases responsiveness to IL-12 [62] which acts via STAT4 leading to proliferation, activation and perforin expression [63]. In the NK cell line NK92, IL-18 stimulates STAT3 signaling [64]. Also further IL-2 family cytokines, such as IL-21 and IL-27, use JAK1, JAK3, STAT1, STAT3, STAT4 and STAT5 for NK cell activation [65, 66]. It can, thus, be expected that factors are present in the decidua, which reduce availability of these signaling molecules in uterine NK cells in order to protect the fetus from maternal NK cell attacks.

Conclusion

The literature provides a multitude of information about the JAK/STAT pathway in lymphocytes, but thus far, very little is known about this system in decidual lymphocytes. JAK/STAT is involved in the differentiation of T helper cells into Th1 and Th2 subsets. Many cytokines signal via this pathway and influence it. Also the production of numerous cytokines and other factors depends on JAK/STAT signaling. It may, therefore, be suggested that the regulation of the JAK/STAT system is crucial for the development and maintenance of the immunological balance in the decidua and placenta necessary for successful pregnancy.

Acknowledgment

Several authors of this manuscript are members of an European Network of Excellence, entitled 'EMBIC' (Embryo Implantation Control), supported by the European Union (contract no. 512040).

References

1 Kamat BR, Isaacson PG: The immunocytochemical distribution of leukocytic subpopulations in human endometrium. Am J Pathol 1987;127:66–73.
2 Kammerer U, von Wolff M, Markert UR: Immunology of human endometrium. Immunobiology 2004;209:569–574.
3 Dietl J, Ruck P, Horny HP, Handgretinger R, Marzusch K, Ruck M, Kaiserling E, Griesser H, Kabelitz D: The decidua of early human pregnancy: Immunohistochemistry and function of immunocompetent cells. Gynecol Obstet Invest 1992;33:197–204.
4 Ihle JN, Nosaka T, Thierfelder W, Quelle FW, Shimoda K: Jaks and Stats in cytokine signaling. Stem Cells 1997;15(suppl 1):105–112.
5 Fung MM, Rohwer F, McGuire KL: IL-2 activation of a PI3K-dependent STAT3 serine phosphorylation pathway in primary human T cells. Cell Signal 2003;15:625–636.
6 Karnitz LM, Abraham RT: Cytokine receptor signaling mechanisms. Curr Opin Immunol 1995; 7:320–326.
7 Nair JS, DaFonseca CJ, Tjernberg A, Sun W, Darnell JE Jr, Chait BT, Zhang JJ: Requirement of Ca^{2+} and CaMKII for Stat1 Ser-727 phosphorylation in response to IFN-gamma. Proc Natl Acad Sci USA 2002;99:5971–5976.
8 Hibi M, Hirano T: Signal transduction through cytokine receptors. Int Rev Immunol 1998;17: 75–102.
9 Leonard WJ, O'Shea JJ: Jaks and STATs: Biological implications. Annu Rev Immunol 1998;16: 293–322.
10 Liu KD, Gaffen SL, Goldsmith MA: JAK/STAT signaling by cytokine receptors. Curr Opin Immunol 1998;10:271–278.
11 Plaetinck G, Combe MC, Corthesy P, Sperisen P, Kanamori H, Honjo T, Nabholz M: Control of IL-2 receptor-alpha expression by IL-1, tumor necrosis factor, and IL-2. Complex regulation via elements in the 5′ flanking region. J Immunol 1990;145:3340–3347.

12 Rusterholz C, Henrioud PC, Nabholz M: Interleukin-2 (IL-2) regulates the accessibility of the IL-2-responsive enhancer in the IL-2 receptor alpha gene to transcription factors. Mol Cell Biol 1999; 19:2681–2689.
13 Osman I, Young A, Ledingham MA, Thomson AJ, Jordan F, Greer IA, Norman JE: Leukocyte density and pro-inflammatory cytokine expression in human fetal membranes, decidua, cervix and myometrium before and during labour at term. Mol Hum Reprod 2003;9:41–45.
14 Chaouat G, Zourbas S, Ostojic S, Lappree-Delage G, Dubanchet S, Ledee N, Martal J: A brief review of recent data on some cytokine expressions at the materno-foetal interface which might challenge the classical Th1/Th2 dichotomy. J Reprod Immunol 2002;53:241–256.
15 Zourbas S, Dubanchet S, Martal J, Chaouat G: Localization of pro-inflammatory (IL-12, IL-15) and anti-inflammatory (IL-11, IL-13) cytokines at the foetomaternal interface during murine pregnancy. Clin Exp Immunol 2001;126:519–528.
16 Lin H, Mosmann TR, Guilbert L, Tuntipopipat S, Wegmann TG: Synthesis of T helper 2-type cytokines at the maternal-fetal interface. J Immunol 1993;151:4562–4573.
17 Wegmann TG, Lin H, Guilbert L, Mosmann TR: Bidirectional cytokine interactions in the maternal-fetal relationship: Is successful pregnancy a TH2 phenomenon? Immunol Today 1993;14:353–356.
18 Piccinni MP, Romagnani S: Regulation of fetal allograft survival by a hormone-controlled Th1- and Th2-type cytokines. Immunol Res 1996;15:141–150.
19 Shuai K, Ziemiecki A, Wilks AF, Harpur AG, Sadowski HB, Gilman MZ, Darnell JE: Polypeptide signalling to the nucleus through tyrosine phosphorylation of Jak and Stat proteins. Nature 1993; 366:580–583.
20 Agnello D, Lankford CS, Bream J, Morinobu A, Gadina M, O'Shea JJ, Frucht DM: Cytokines and transcription factors that regulate T helper cell differentiation: New players and new insights. J Clin Immunol 2003;23:147–161.
21 Makhseed M, Raghupathy R, El-Shazly S, Azizieh F, Al-Harmi JA, Al-Azemi MM: Pro-inflammatory maternal cytokine profile in preterm delivery. Am J Reprod Immunol 2003;49: 308–318.
22 El-Shazly S, Makhseed M, Azizieh F, Raghupathy R: Increased expression of pro-inflammatory cytokines in placentas of women undergoing spontaneous preterm delivery or premature rupture of membranes. Am J Reprod Immunol 2004;52:45–52.
23 Szekeres-Bartho J, Wegmann TG: A progesterone-dependent immunomodulatory protein alters the Th1/Th2 balance. J Reprod Immunol 1996;31:81–95.
24 Joachim R, Zenclussen AC, Polgar B, Douglas AJ, Fest S, Knackstedt M, Klapp BF, Arck PC: The progesterone derivative dydrogesterone abrogates murine stress-triggered abortion by inducing a Th2 biased local immune response. Steroids 2003;68:931–940.
25 Paul WE: Interleukin 4: Signalling mechanisms and control of T cell differentiation. Ciba Found Symp 1997;204:208–219.
26 Yu CR, Young HA, Ortaldo JR: Characterization of cytokine differential induction of STAT complexes in primary human T and NK cells. J Leukoc Biol 1998;64:245–258.
27 Stamm LM, Raisanen-Sokolowski A, Okano M, Russell ME, David JR, Satoskar AR: Mice with STAT6-targeted gene disruption develop a Th1 response and control cutaneous leishmaniasis. J Immunol 1998;161:6180–6188.
28 Smeltz RB, Chen J, Hu-Li J, Shevach EM: Regulation of interleukin (IL)-18 receptor alpha chain expression on CD4(+) T cells during T helper (Th)1/Th2 differentiation. Critical downregulatory role of IL-4. J Exp Med 2001;194:143–153.
29 Yu CR, Kirken RA, Malabarba MG, Young HA, Ortaldo JR: Differential regulation of the Janus kinase-STAT pathway and biologic function of IL-13 in primary human NK and T cells: A comparative study with IL-4. J Immunol 1998;161:218–227.
30 Chaouat G, Assal Meliani A, Martal J, Raghupathy R, Elliot J, Mosmann T, Wegmann TG: IL-10 prevents naturally occurring fetal loss in the CBA × DBA/2 mating combination, and local defect in IL-10 production in this abortion-prone combination is corrected by in vivo injection of IFN-tau. J Immunol 1995;154:4261–4268.
31 Kotenko SV, Pestka S: Jak-Stat signal transduction pathway through the eyes of cytokine class II receptor complexes. Oncogene 2000;19:2557–2565.

32 Dumoutier L, Lejeune D, Hor S, Fickenscher H, Renauld JC: Cloning of a new type II cytokine receptor activating signal transducer and activator of transcription (STAT)1, STAT2 and STAT3. Biochem J 2003;370:391–396.

33 Williams L, Bradley L, Smith A, Foxwell B: Signal transducer and activator of transcription 3 is the dominant mediator of the anti-inflammatory effects of IL-10 in human macrophages. J Immunol 2004;172:567–576.

34 Wang M, Liang P: Interleukin-24 and its receptors. Immunology 2005;114:166–170.

35 Murphy KM, Reiner SL: The lineage decisions of helper T cells. Nat Rev Immunol 2002; 2:933–944.

36 Frucht DM, Aringer M, Galon J, Danning C, Brown M, Fan S, Centola M, Wu CY, Yamada N, El Gabalawy H, O'Shea JJ: Stat4 is expressed in activated peripheral blood monocytes, dendritic cells, and macrophages at sites of Th1-mediated inflammation. J Immunol 2000;164:4659–4664.

37 Muthian G, Bright JJ: Quercetin, a flavonoid phytoestrogen, ameliorates experimental allergic encephalomyelitis by blocking IL-12 signaling through JAK-STAT pathway in T lymphocyte. J Clin Immunol 2004;24:542–552.

38 Li-Weber M: TH1/TH2. Mod Asp Immunobiol 2003;3:46.

39 Wurtz O, Bajenoff M, Guerder S: IL-4-mediated inhibition of IFN-gamma production by CD4+ T cells proceeds by several developmentally regulated mechanisms. Int Immunol 2004;16:501–508.

40 Wilson R, Jenkins C, Miller H, McInnes IB, Moore J, McLean MA, Walker JJ: Abnormal cytokine levels in non-pregnant women with a history of recurrent miscarriage. Eur J Obstet Gynecol Reprod Biol 2004;115:51–54.

41 Kilic M, Flossmann E, Flossmann O, Vogelsang H, Junker U, Chaouat G, Markert UR: Jeg-3 human choriocarcinoma-induced immunosuppression: Downregulation of interleukin-2, interleukin-2 receptor alpha-chain, and its Jak/Stat signaling pathway. Am J Reprod Immunol 1999; 41:61–69.

42 Wang KS, Ritz J, Frank DA: IL-2 induces STAT4 activation in primary NK cells and NK cell lines, but not in T cells. J Immunol 1999;162:299–304.

43 Benczik M, Gaffen SL: The interleukin (IL)-2 family cytokines: Survival and proliferation signaling pathways in T lymphocytes. Immunol Invest 2004;33:109–142.

44 Markert UR, Kilic M, Schleussner E, Vogelsang H: Choriocarcinoma-induced suppression of lymphocyte activity. J Investig Allergol Clin Immunol 2000;10:323–326.

45 Wang H, Xie X, Lu WG, Ye DF, Chen HZ, Li X, Cheng Q: Ovarian carcinoma cells inhibit T cell proliferation: Suppression of IL-2 receptor beta and gamma expression and their JAK-STAT signaling pathway. Life Sci 2004;74:1739–1749.

46 Storl F: Einfluss von Trophoblastzellen auf die Interleukinproduktion, Rezeptorexpression und intrazelluläre Signaltransduktion allogener Lymphozyten; dissertation, Jena, 2004.

47 Eriksen KW, Sommer VH, Woetmann A, Rasmussen AB, Brender C, Svejgaard A, Skov S, Geisler C, Odum N: Bi-phasic effect of interferon (IFN)-alpha: IFN-alpha up- and down-regulates interleukin-4 signaling in human T cells. J Biol Chem 2004;279:169–176.

48 Paulesu L, Bocci V, King A, Loke YM: Immunocytochemical localization of interferons in human trophoblast populations. J Biol Regul Homeost Agents 1991;5:81–85.

49 Gamero AM, Sakamoto S, Montenegro J, Larner AC: Identification of a novel conserved motif in the STAT family that is required for tyrosine phosphorylation. J Biol Chem 2004; 279:12379–12385.

50 Strengell M, Julkunen I, Matikainen S: IFN-alpha regulates IL-21 and IL-21R expression in human NK and T cells. J Leukoc Biol 2004;76:416–422.

51 Yu CR, Mahdi RM, Ebong S, Vistica BP, Chen J, Guo Y, Gery I, Egwuagu CE: Cell proliferation and STAT6 pathways are negatively regulated in T cells by STAT1 and suppressors of cytokine signaling. J Immunol 2004;173:737–746.

52 Anderson P, Sundstedt A, Li L, O'Neill EJ, Li S, Wraith DC, Wang P: Differential activation of signal transducer and activator of transcription (STAT)3 and STAT5 and induction of suppressors of cytokine signalling in T(h)1 and T(h)2 cells. Int Immunol 2003;15:1309–1317.

53 Yamamoto K, Yamaguchi M, Miyasaka N, Miura O: SOCS-3 inhibits IL-12-induced STAT4 activation by binding through its SH2 domain to the STAT4 docking site in the IL-12 receptor beta2 subunit. Biochem Biophys Res Commun 2003;310:1188–1193.

54 Fujimoto M, Tsutsui H, Yumikura-Futatsugi S, Ueda H, Xingshou O, Abe T, Kawase I, Nakanishi K, Kishimoto T, Naka T: A regulatory role for suppressor of cytokine signaling-1 in T(h) polarization in vivo. Int Immunol 2002;14:1343–1350.
55 Blumenstein M, Bowen-Shauver JM, Keelan JA, Mitchell MD: Identification of suppressors of cytokine signaling (SOCS) proteins in human gestational tissues: Differential regulation is associated with the onset of labor. J Clin Endocrinol Metab 2002;87:1094–1097.
56 Keelan JA, Blumenstein M, Helliwell RJ, Sato TA, Marvin KW, Mitchell MD: Cytokines, prostaglandins and parturition – a review. Placenta 2003;24(suppl A):S33–S46.
57 Gubbay O, Critchley HO, Bowen JM, King A, Jabbour HN: Prolactin induces ERK phosphorylation in epithelial and CD56(+) natural killer cells of the human endometrium. J Clin Endocrinol Metab 2002;87:2329–2335.
58 Barkai U, Prigent-Tessier A, Tessier C, Gibori GB, Gibori G: Involvement of SOCS-1, the suppressor of cytokine signaling, in the prevention of prolactin-responsive gene expression in decidual cells. Mol Endocrinol 2000;14:554–563.
59 Sun R, Li AL, Wei HM, Tian ZG: Expression of prolactin receptor and response to prolactin stimulation of human NK cell lines. Cell Res 2004;14:67–73.
60 Zhang J, Sun R, Wei H, Tian Z: Antitumor effects of recombinant human prolactin in human adenocarcinoma-bearing SCID mice with human NK cell xenograft. Int Immunopharmacol 2005; 5:417–425.
61 Ashkar AA, Di Santo JP, Croy BA: Interferon gamma contributes to initiation of uterine vascular modification, decidual integrity, and uterine natural killer cell maturation during normal murine pregnancy. J Exp Med 2000;192:259–270.
62 Wang KS, Frank DA, Ritz J: Interleukin-2 enhances the response of natural killer cells to interleukin-12 through up-regulation of the interleukin-12 receptor and STAT4. Blood 2000; 95: 3183–3190.
63 Yamamoto K, Shibata F, Miyasaka N, Miura O: The human perforin gene is a direct target of STAT4 activated by IL-12 in NK cells. Biochem Biophys Res Commun 2002;297:1245–1252.
64 Kalina U, Kauschat D, Koyama N, Nuernberger H, Ballas K, Koschmieder S, Bug G, Hofmann WK, Hoelzer D, Ottmann OG: IL-18 activates STAT3 in the natural killer cell line 92, augments cytotoxic activity, and mediates IFN-gamma production by the stress kinase p38 and by the extracellular regulated kinases p44erk-1 and p42erk-21. J Immunol 2000;165:1307–1313.
65 Lucas S, Ghilardi N, Li J, de Sauvage FJ: IL-27 regulates IL-12 responsiveness of naive CD4+ T cells through Stat1-dependent and -independent mechanisms. Proc Natl Acad Sci USA 2003; 100:15047–15052.
66 Habib T, Nelson A, Kaushansky K: IL-21: A novel IL-2-family lymphokine that modulates B, T, and natural killer cell responses. J Allergy Clin Immunol 2003;112:1033–1045.

PD Dr. Udo R. Markert
Abteilung für Geburtshilfe
Friedrich-Schiller-Universität
DE–07740 Jena (Germany)
Tel. +49 3641 933763, Fax +49 3641 933764
E-Mail markert@med.uni-jena.de

Market UR (ed): Immunology of Pregnancy.
Chem Immunol Allergy. Basel, Karger, 2005, vol 89, pp 36–48

Tolerance Signaling Molecules

David A. Clark

McMaster University, Hamilton, Canada

Abstract

Mechanisms explaining maternal tolerance of her semiallogeneic histoincompatible fetus have been proposed to include a number of unique signaling molecules including CD200, novel MHC class I-b molecules such as HLA-G and HLA-E, Th2,3 cytokines, apoptosis-inducing molecules such as FASL, and indoleamine 2,3-dioxygenase. Novel CD4+CD25+ Treg cells and γδ T cell receptor-positive regulatory cells appear to play key roles in responding to and in generating signals. This chapter will critically review current data concerning the mechanisms and relevance of the various proposed mechanisms.

Introduction

In the beginning, the purpose of the immune system was to distinguish self from nonself, and to reject nonself [1]. Not to tolerate self was a real 'horror autotoxicus' (Ehrlich) that led to autoimmune diseases. Not to tolerate self also leads to other unpleasant consequences. For example, the gut is full of food antigens and commensal bacteria. Reacting to absorbed food antigens (and/or bacterial antigens) could cause both local and systemic inflammation. Similarly, inhaled antigens in air could cause asthma and pulmonary inflammatory conditions. At a related mucosal surface, the vagina and uterus, reactions to male tissue antigens (e.g. spermatozoa, seminal plasma) and to male antigens expressed by the embryo could abrogate reproductive processes essential to survival of an outbred species. In this chapter I am not going to review *all* of the details explaining how the immune system is organized to ensure health rather than disease. Instead, I will discuss some key signaling mechanisms promoting 'tolerance' of nonself antigens and the key issue of ensuring pregnancy success when the implanted embryo is 'normal' and needed.

Tolerance Concepts

The conventional view of antigen-specific 'tolerance' is primarily centered on activation versus nonactivation of antigen-specific thymus-derived (T) cells bearing conventional αβ receptors for antigen (TcR). Here, antigen, usually in the from of 9 amino acid peptides, are 'presented' in the groove of a class MHC class I or MHC class II self-antigen by antigen-presenting cells (APC) such as dendritic cells or macrophages. Triggering of the T cells requires binding of CD4 on T cells to class II MHC or CD8 on the T cells to class I to complete 'signal 1', followed by costimulation provided by binding of CD80/86 to CD288 on the T cell or CD40L to CD40 along with additional adhesion interactions mediated by ICAM1,2,3 with LFA-1 (on the T cell) or LFA-3 (on the APC) with CD2 on the T cell. Expansion of the activated T cell was then facilitated by growth factors (cytokines) provided by the APC and/or T cell itself. T cells making proinflammatory cytokines such as IL-2, TNF-α, IFN-γ, and related mediators (IL-12, IL-15, IL-18) promoted cell-mediated immune rejection. Cytokines such as IL-3, IL-4, IL-6, IL-10, IL-13 (called Th2 as distinct from Th1) promoted antibody production by antigen-activated B cells, and antibody then promoted humoral rejection. In this model, 'tolerance' could occur due to ignorance, anergy, clonal deletion (apoptosis/exhaustion), or regulation.

'Ignorance' could occur due to a lack of antigen presentation, or absence of T cells with receptors for that particular peptide + MHC combination. The latter represents holes in the repertoire occurring as T cell mature in the thymus where T cells first expand in response to self-MHC, and then cells reactive with self-MHC and self-MHC-bearing self-peptides are vetoed. A hole in the repertoire occurred when T cells able to react with certain foreign antigen + self-MHC did not develop. Absence CD4 or CD8 could also prevent effective binding of TcR to antigen. 'Anergy', on the other hand, could arise following binding to TcR to antigen if one or more of the important second signals were missing. An alternative consequence of missing second signals could be activation of pathways leading to apoptosis. T cells becoming apoptotic were then deleted. 'Regulation' on the other hand represented a distinct mechanism where outsiders (e.g. regulatory T cells) acted to stop an ongoing immune response or to stop it at the outset. Self-tolerance preventing autoimmunity has been ascribed in mice to a distinct population of regulatory CD4+25+ αβ T cells emigrating from thymus in the immediate postnatal period. The mechanism of action of these Treg cells is debated. Direct cell contact is required, and cell surface TGF-β, a cytokine that suppresses both Th1 and Th2 response, has been proposed, as well as production of CTLA4. CTLA4 binds to CD80/86 and blocks binding to CD28 on T cells; CTLA4 also reverse signals via CD80/86 such that APC express indoleamine 2,3-dioxygenase (IDO) that deprives nearby activated T cells of tryptophan [2]. Such starvation leads to apoptosis. A novel population of allo-MHC-specific CD4–8– T cells (double-negative or DN cells) can suppress via expression of FASL that binds to FAS receptors on activated CD4 or CD8 Th1 Th2 T cells and causes their apoptosis [3]. Finally, certain populations of regulatory CD4 and CD8 T cells will make TGF-β (and related IL-10 that inhibits Th1 response) when these cells are proliferating in the presence of these cytokines, and CD4+25+ Treg cells may act in part by facilitating expansion of these cytokine-secreting populations [4, 5].

It is important to stress that there is a more primitive immune system, the innate or natural immune system, which is hard-wired to act without a complex activation sequence of αβ T cells and their expansion which delays action, and to act as an immediate defense at the interface between mucosa/skin and the outside world. These cells include macrophages and related APCs, polymorphonuclear leukocytes, natural killer (NK) cells, and mast cells (that produce a variety of mediators and Th1 cytokines). Indeed, the classical antigen-specific immune system depends upon an activated innate system APC to stimulate αβ T cell immunity. Matzinger [6] has suggested that it is danger signals (that are seen by the innate system) that decide if the classical αβ T cell system will react to antigen. Danger signals upregulate expression of costimulatory molecules such as CD80/86 on APC as well as expression of class II MHC that presents peptides to CD4+ T cells. Danger signals such as LPS can also act directly on B cells to produce polyclonal autoantibody responses and autoimmunity. As a certain amount of 'danger' is present at mucosal surfaces and must be tolerated, 'tolerance' mechanisms are also needed.

There are a large number of hard-wired receptors for PAMP danger signals, and currently, the focus is on toll-like (tlr) molecules [7]. Failure to express particular tlrs at an adequate level on the cell surface could potentially recreate the 'ignorance' phenomenon. TGF-β and IL-10 are cytokines that may promote quiescence amongst innate effector cells [8]. NK cells are also turned off via self-MHC interaction with surface KIR (Ly49A-N in the mouse) and/or CD94/NKG2 receptors (and it has been proposed NK cells are hard-wired to react to absent self MHC) [9]. (Some KIR-MHC interactions can activate, and Ly49 subtypes show a degree of MHC specificity.) There is also a population T cells bearing γδ TcR which can arise in part in the absence of a thymus, which accumulate in mucosa and skin, and which can recognize antigens in the absence of MHC and without need for CD4 or CD8 [10]. Some of these γδ T cells when activated become effector cells, but many act as suppressor cells. Interestingly, a significant percentage of γδ TcR+ cells express CD94/NKG2, and a small percentage express KIRs. There are also cells with both T and NK cell markers, both NKαβT cells and NKγδT cells [11]. The αβ type tends to see antigens in the context of atypical MHC class I-b antigens (such as CD1, or

MHC-linked Qa-$1^{a/b}$, Qa-2, TL) [12]. The recognition patterns of innate system cells is therefore distinct from the adaptive αβ T cell system which can see antigen in the context of MHC class I-a, I-b, or II. Another difference is that the adaptive immune system has memory, and will react more rapidly and with a magnified response to a second challenge with antigen, whereas innate system cells lack memory. However, just as an activated innate system facilitates immune responses by the adaptive immune system, the innate system can have suppressive effects on its own activity as well as on the adaptive system. Production of tolerogenic cytokines such as TGF-β provides one mechanism. Certain immunoregulatory APC, primarily dendritic cells, express CD200, a costimulatory molecule that is the antithesis of CD80/86 [13]. APC with CD200 receptors may be downregulated, and γδ T cells exposed to antigen + CD200 may become antigen-specific suppressor cells acting on both the adaptive and innate systems via TGF-β and IL-10 [14].

What does the above have to do with successful reproduction? The conceptus is enveloped in a cocoon of fetal trophoblast cells that form the fetomaternal interface and placenta. Nonreactivity of the conventional αβ T cell system with trophoblast was attributed to lack of expression of classical class I-a and class II paternal MHC, but forced expression of class I-a MHC on trophoblast did not overcome the problem [15]. Although excess paternal class I-a expression could deplete systemic αβ T cells reactive with such antigens [16], the relevance of this phenomenon was questionable as only at the implanting blastocyst stage can αβ T cells harm embryos (via deposition of proinflammatory C3) and only when the local effects of IDO are blocked [17]. By contrast, γδ T cells, specifically the subset expressing Vγ1.1 in the mouse, is able to react with trophoblasts from a variety of species [18]. The cytokine pattern produced by these cells depends on presence or absence of CD200 and Th1 versus Th2/3 cytokines. CD200 and possibly Th2/3 cytokines promote cells which make a novel TGF-$\beta_{2,3}$-type molecule [19]. Conventional TGF-βs, $\beta_{1,2,3}$, have a 25-kDa bioactive form, whereas in both the mouse and human, the γδ suppressor cells in deciduas make a lower molecular weight homodimer, which is relatively less fibrogenic for its immunosuppressive potency [20, 21]. Another innate immune effector, the NK cell, has been implicated in 'rejection' of embryos at a later stage of gestation when a distinct fetus and placenta have developed (e.g. the CBA × DBA/2 model), but must act indirectly as there is no evidence trophoblast cells (with or without paternal MHC expression) are killed, and the relevant abortogenic cells are not graft rejecting TcRdβ T cells but are NK cells probably coexpressing Vγ1.1 and are thus NKγδT cells [22, 23]. The importance of 'danger' signals also merits emphasis. The CBA × DBA/2 system is a novel mating where there is a lack of maternal NKγδT cell tolerance to an as yet undefined paternal antigen [24]. Abortions are promoted by Th1 cytokines, flora/LPS, and stress that enhances gut permeability (and LPS absorption). In most mouse mating systems, including natural matings in the wild, more heterozygous allogeneic embryos have a survival advantage compared to homozygous (more syngeneic) embryos [25]. This has been attributed to activation of protective suppressor cells by more foreign/allogeneic embryos to facilitate birth of progeny more likely to survive in a dangerous (e.g. stressful) environment. Indeed, in the CBA × DBA/2 model, a specific non-MHC antigen presented in the context of paternal MHC-linked antigens protects [24], BALB/c can prime for a protective response [26], and there is new information concerning the identity of the protective T cell subsets in the uterus and how they may act.

In the remainder of this chapter, I will discuss four types of putative tolerance signaling molecules and how they may facilitate fetomaternal tolerance to enhance the chance of survival of heterozygous embryos.

CD200-CD200R Interaction

CD200 is a glycoprotein which lacks a transmembrane signaling domain and must act by binding to a receptor [13]. There are four CD200 receptor subtypes described [27]. Current antibodies do not distinguish between CD200R1 and R4, so these will be denoted as CD200R1/4. In the murine uterus, all CD200R subtypes are expressed, but R1/4 and R3 are most evident, and are seen on trophoblast cells and in certain areas of the deciduas on days 8.5–12.5 of pregnancy. R2 is also expressed [28].

The relevance of CD200 for reproduction was originally suspected when CD200 was found essential for induction of alloantigen-specific tolerance to kidney allografts [14]. Portal vein infusion of donor splenocytes induced CD4–8– γδTs that activated via cytokines such as TGF-β and IL-10 [14]. As such, these γδTs were very similar to the cells found in the decidua of successful allogeneic pregnancies in mice [20]. In situ hybridization for CD200 mRNA demonstrated expression on fetal trophoblast and in certain areas of deciduas (a cap at the peripheral margin of the primary deciduas and in the mesometrial secondary decidual zone) [29]. The functional significance of CD200 and its receptors was then obtained by use of anti-CD200-neutralizing monoclonal antibody and by injection of a soluble immunosuppressiveCD200Fc construct using the abortion-prone CBA × DBA/2 model. In this model, it was known that expression of fgl2 prothrombinase triggered losses by activating inflammation via thrombin generation [22, 29]. The abortion rate was about 40–50% of that expected on the basis of implantations overexpressing fgl2. The expected rate of loss was achieved when monoclonal anti-CD200 was injected. A single dose on gestation day 8.5 or 9.5 was more effective than treatment on gestation day 7.5, and CD200Fc given on day 8.5 reduced the abortion rate to <4% [29]. Abortion rates in CBA × BALB/c matings (where the striking accumulation of Th1 NKγδT cells from gestation day 5.5 is not seen [30]) were also increased by anti-CD200 antibody, suggesting a continuing role of CD200-CD200R interaction was required from day 8.5 of pregnancy to prevent abortions.

Interestingly, administration of BALB/c splenocytes to CBA females was known to prevent abortions in the CBA × DBA/2 model, and a prior pregnancy by BALB/c protected similarly [26]. The BALB/c splenocytes were effective if given before pregnancy, or during early pregnancy up to day 7.5 of pregnancy (although the progesterone-induced release of an NK blocking factor was able to act on day 8.5–10.5), and CD8α+ cells were required to mediate suppression as was also the case when GM-CSF was used to prevent abortions [31]. Further, blocking CD200 on the BALB/c splenocytes abrogated suppression [32]. As BALB/c cells survive for a period of time following injection, it was puzzling why the CD200+ cells did not show the protective effect that was seen when CD200Fc was injected on day 8.5 or 9.5 of gestation. Obviously, the answer had to lie in the mechanism. The effect of CD200Fc is most likely pharmacological and acts on CD200R on cells which have either 'seen' antigen or do not 'see' antigen. CD200R is expressed on trophoblast and other cells in decidua, most likely APC and γδT cells [28]. In contrast, the effect of action of CD200+ splenocytes is likely mediated by immunogenic APC, such as BALB/c *dendritic* cells. The protective antigen on BALB/c has been studied using (DBA/2 × BALB/c) × DBA/2 recombinant lines. Two nonallelic minor antigens denoted as P (protects against abortion) and S (stimulates abortion) were identified. P appears to be a peptide (i.e. minor histocompatibility antigen) expressed by both DBA/2 and BALB/c which must be expressed in the context of MHC H-2^d [24]. The MHC antigen required is probably not MHC class I-a (H-2K, L, or D), but rather the class I-b antigen Qa-2 is essential: Qa-2 is known to be expressed on mouse embryo cells and trophoblasts. BALB/c sublines expressing low Qa-2 compared to BALB/cJ were unable to immunize CBA/J females against abortions when mated with DBA/2 males. The S antigen, by contrast, appeared to be expressed in DBA/2, and is therefore not likely MHC H-2^d restricted. This is important as cells with TcR γδ can recognize class I-b MHC and other small molecules, but not peptides bound in the groove of an MHC molecule [12, 33]. It would be possible for Th1 NKγδT and Th1 γδ T cells to react to S, but not to P. The minor antigen P peptide could, however, be recognized by αβ TcR+ cells. There is a striking accumulation of TcR αβ+ T cells in the secondary decidua of CBA × DBA/2 matings on gestation day 5.5 when APC such as macrophages are infiltrating [22, 30]. If these T cells were stimulated by soluble P peptide associated with Qa-2, generation of a regulatory environment with Th2 cytokine production should bias differentiation of activated γδ T cells towards the Th2/3 phenotype [19]. Thus, CD4+25+ Treg cells may play an important role in local γδ T cell differentiation. Adoptive transfer of CD4+25+ Treg cells from the spleens of day 14.5 CBA × BALB/c mated mice to CBA × DBA/2 mated mice on gestation day 0.5 or 1.5 or 2.5 (but not thereafter) has recently been reported to present abortions [34]. Treg cells also infiltrate deciduas at the implantation site in other mating combinations, and removal of the CD25+ subset of CD4+ T cells appears to result in a combination of classical resorptions and early occult pregnancy failure [35]. As CD4+25+ Treg cells require IL-2 to develop, and no IL-2 has been found in decidua [4], Treg production is likely systemic rather than local. Alternately, Treg cells may have a different growth factor receptor and ligand.

Our understanding of S and P and related tolerance signaling molecules would be greatly enhanced if the S and P molecules were cloned, and subtractive hybridization using the most extreme of the recombinant lines has been considered [24]. Vγ1.1+ TcR+ cells can react to all trophoblasts, including within-species and extra-species xenogeneic trophoblasts [18]. Is S the antigen, or is S a peptide that interferes with P? Where do CD200Fc and CD200+ alloantigenic BALB/c cells act, and via which CD200Rs? CD200R1/4 signaling may lead to direct suppression whereas preliminary data suggests CD200R2 or R3 signaling may act via CD4+25+ cell activation as the Th1?Th2 cytokine shift is much less [27, 28]. Are the CD8α+ suppressor cells required for amelioration of abortion in CBA × DBA/2 matings and for additional abortion reduction in response to BALB/c splenocyte treatment CD8+ αβ Ts cells that make Th2 cytokines impacting γδ T cell development, or are they CD8αα+ dendritic cells expressing CD200 [36]? Which of the immunoprotective responses occur locally in decidua, and which occur systemically? Reduction in CD200 expression has proven essential for fgl2 prothrombinase triggering of abortions, but the mechanisms of this suppression remain hypothetical [29]. It is known that a 'danger' signal acting via tlr is required along with the Th1 cytokines TNF-α and IFN-γ [37]. Finally, CD200 and CD200Rs are expressed both in decidua and in trophoblasts. Are both sites important? Does CD200 have effects other than immunoregulation of CD200R+ trophoblast cells? Many questions, and as yet, no answers.

What about Atypical Class I-b Molecules such as HLA-G and HLA-E?

Although trophoblasts prior to implantation downregulate cell surface expression of most class I-a and class II molecules, certain class I-b molecules and paternal minor histocompatibility antigens are expressed, albeit sometimes in soluble form. Table 1 summarizes similarities and differences between the mouse and human. HLA-G was found to inhibit cytotoxicity by NK cells, and thought important given the presence of atypical CD16– NK cells in the decidua of successful pregnancies and increased presence of classical CD16+ NK cells in pregnancy failure [22]. It has been argued that Qa-2 may be the homolog of human HLA-G1 and G2 [41] but recently another mouse homolog of HLA-G1 and G2 called blastocyst antigens 1 and 2 (BA1 and 2) has been reported [42]. Production of soluble HLA-G may be essential for implantation [44], but some HLA-G-deficient humans (but perhaps not all [45]) reproduce successfully, and the CBA × DBA/2 and CBA × BALB/c systems lack expression of the murine HLA-G1 and G2 analogs BA1 and BA2 [42]; on the other hand, blocking IL-10 increases abortions in CBA × BALB/c matings and this IL-10 dependence is not seen in other mating combinations where the murine analogs of human HLA-G1 and G2 exist [41, 46]. It is also possible to prevent abortions in the CBA × DBA/2 model by injecting L cells transfected with H-2L [47], so MHC-dependent inhibition of NK, and NK$\gamma\delta$T cells could represent an antiabortive mechanism. However, this protective effect of transfected cells may represent a pharmacological effect that does not occur physiologically. HLA-G in the human is thought to facilitate expression of HLA-E (homologous to murine Qa-1^b which has *not* been described on embryo trophoblast), and HLA-E inhibits NK cell cytotoxicity [43]. However, there is no evidence that NK cells act via direct perforin-mediated cytotoxicity to cause abortions. Indeed, perforin knockout mice can abort [48]! NK and related innate effector cells act via their cytokine production, and the role of MHC-KIR and MHC-CD94/NKG2 interactions does not appear to fit the Th1/Th2 paradigm [49].

Recently it has been shown that HLA-G expression may promote survival of allografts [50]. Such data suggest HLA-G could play a role in semiallogeneic pregnancy success, but more convincing data is required.

What about Apoptosis-Inducing Molecules?

One mechanism of tolerance described above is inactivation of effector cells via induction of apoptosis. As mentioned, DN $\alpha\beta$ FASL+ Ts cells have been described in one model of allograft tolerance using the class I-a MHC H-2L [3]. It was suggested by Hunt et al. [51] that mice deficient in FASL might experience reproductive failure. This was not found reproducible by Rogers et al. [52], and Chaouat and Clark [53] found no evident problems with FAS– mice even when the female was preimmunized against paternal antigens. The poor reproductive performance in the study of Hunt et al. was most likely an artifact related to conditions in her animal colony (e.g. excess 'danger'). Other

Table 1. Comparison of expression of different types of antigens by trophoblasts in mice and humans

Species	MHC class I-a	MHC class I-b	Minor H antigens
Mouse	H-2 [16, 22, 39]	Qa-2 [41], BA1 and 2 [42], Qa-1[a]	yes [15]
Human	HLA-C [3, 8, 40]	HLA-G1 and G2 [40], HLA-E [43]	?

[a]Not reported to be expressed by trophoblasts.

apoptosis-inducing lined-receptor combinations have been suggested as alternatives to FASL-FAS (e.g. trail), but no in vivo evidence has been forthcoming. Indeed, there are so many apoptosis-inducing pathways, it may not be possible to conduct a convincing scientific experiment (as defined by Popper), as *all* apoptosis pathways would have to be blocked to abrogate 'tolerance' [24]. Chaouat and Clark [53] did note higher levels of antifetal CTL in the spleens of allopregnant FAS– females, so FAS-FASL might provide a mechanism for females to dispose of antigen-fetal cells escaping into her circulation during pregnancy.

What about IDO?

The immunosuppressive effects of IDO on alloreactive αβ T cells has been described above. Mellor et al. [17] reported that blocking IDO by administration of 1-methyl-tryptophan caused CD4+ maternal T cells to accumulate in deciduas and cause pregnancy failure via deposition of the C3 component of complement. These losses began within 2 days after implantation in mice, and before the formation of a distinct fetus and placenta when classical abortions (resorptions) occur [54]. The losses were allospecific and paternal minor antigens as well as MHC played a role [17]. The phenomenon was similar to rejection of allogeneic blastocysts placed under the kidney capsule of mice preimmunized to minor paternal transplantation antigens; by contrast, trophoblasts developing later in gestation were not rejectable [15]. Similar early losses (equivalent to occult loss or chemical pregnancies in humans) was producible by injecting monoclonal antibody H57 that binds to TcR α and activates αβ T cells, and by α-GalCer that activates NKαβT cells via a CD1-dependent process [30, 55]. In the latter model, it was proven that perforin was required [55]. These early loss models are quite distinct from the spontaneous abortion models and IDO+ cells are viewed as essential for 'tolerance' that prevents rejection of the 'fetal allograft'. There are IDO+ APC in deciduas, and possibly trophoblasts can produce IDO although direct evidence is hard to find; since αβ T cells do not react to trophoblasts, there may be no need for IDO here.

Recently occult loss in the A/J × DBA/2 model has been studied to determine if stress might cause loss by inhibiting expression of IDO [56]. To our surprise, stress-induced occult losses occurred without reduced IDO in deciduas, but Th1/Th2 ratios were increased. Alloimmunization reduced IDO, which is what one would expect if the immune response were to be able to proceed; occult loss in this setting was entirely consistent with the increase in decidual Th1/Th2 ratios. Indeed, combined treatment produced quite low IDO levels and higher Th1/Th2 ratios, but no increase in the rate of occult loss. A similar limitation has been observed in the CBA × DBA/2 abortion model and has been explained by the need for an adequate level of 'danger' signals (e.g. LPS) absorbed from the intestine. LPS can also cause occult loss [37]! Taken together, these observations suggest that occult losses, like abortions, are caused by the combined action of Th1 cytokines and a danger signal in the absence of counteracting Th2/3 cytokines. The purpose is to terminate pregnancy, a burden, when the health and life of the mother are in jeopardy. In this situation, heterozygous embryos are less likely to be lost, as shown by Potts et al. [25]. If reduced IDO were the mechanism of pregnancy termination, one would have the selective elimination of the more heterozygous (antigenic) embryos. Indeed, in a poly-IC-induced loss model where poly-IC acts via tlr3, the loss rate of syngeneic matings was much greater than of allogeneic matings [44, 57]. (The higher abortion rate in the CBA × DBA/2 model is an anomaly due to an NKγδT cell reaction driven by the S signal.) One situation in which loss due to low IDO might prove advantageous would be elimination of chromosomally abnormal embryos. Here, rejection would benefit the mother and the species. Some preliminary human data may support this hypothesis, but further work will be needed to determine if IDO has any significance to naturally occurring reproductive pathology such as recurrent loss of karyotype-normal embryos, or rather, is merely an artifact of a model in which IDO can be completely inhibited pharmacologically (>5 mg of 1-methyltryptophan per mouse per day was required for any effect [17]).

References

1 Janeway CA, Travers P, Walput M, Shomchik MJ: Immunology, ed 6. New York, Garland, 2005.

2 Munn DH, Sharma MD, Mellor AL: Ligation of B7–1/B7–2 by human CD4+ T cells triggers indoleamine 2,3-dioxygenase activity in dendritic cells. J Immunol 2004;172:4100–4110.

3 Zhang ZX, Yang L, Young KJ, DuTemple B, Zhang L: Identification of a previously unknown antigen-specific regulatory T cell and its mechanism of suppression. Nat Med 2000;6:782–789.

4 Nelson BH: IL-2, regulatory T cells, and tolerance. J Immunol 2004;172:3983–3988.

5 Stassen M, Fondel S, Bopp T, Richer C, Muller C, Kubach J, Becker C, Knop J, Enk AH, Schmitt S, Schmitt E, Jonuleit H: Human CD25+ regulatory T cells: Two subsets defined by the integrins $\alpha 4\beta 7$ or $\alpha 4\beta 1$ confer distinct suppressive properties on CD4+ T helper cells. Eur J Immunol 2004;34:1303–1311.
6 Matzinger P: Tolerance, danger, and the extended family. Annu Rev Immunol 1994;12:991–1045.
7 Jeffries C, O'Neil LAJ: Signal transduction pathways activated by toll-like receptors. Mod Asp Immunobiol 2002;2:169–175.
8 Kehlen A, Geisler M, Olsen J, Sablotzki A, Langner J, Reimann D: IL-10 and TGF-β differ in their regulation of aminopeptidase N/CD13 expression in monocytes. Int J Mol Med 2004;13:877–882.
9 Middleton D, Curran M, Maxwell L: Natural killer cells and their receptors. Transplant Immunol 2002;10:147–164.
10 Hayday A, Tigelaar R: Immunoregulation in the tissues by γδ T cells. Nat Rev Immunol 2003; 3:233–242.
11 van Beneden K, Stevenaert F, Leclercq G: Role of inhibitory NK receptors controlling thymic differentiation and functional activity of TCR Vγ3 lymphocytes. Mol Asp Immunobiol 2002; 2:261–264.
12 Shawar SM, Vyas JM, Rodgers JR, Rich RR: Antigen presentation by major histocompatibility complex class I-B molecules. Annu Rev Immunol 1994;12:839–880.
13 Ragheb R, Abrahams S, Beecroft R, Hu J, Ni J, Ramakrishna V, Yu G, Gorczynski RM: Preparation and functional properties of monoclonal antibodies to human, mouse and rat OX-2. Immunol Lett 1999;68:311–315.
14 Gorczynski RM, Cohen Z, Leung Y, Chen Z: γδ TCR+ hybridomas derived from mice perimmunized via the portal vein adoptively transfer increased skin allograft survival. J Immunol 1996; 157:574–581.
15 Clark DA: Controversies in reproductive immunology. Crit Rev Immunol 1991;11:215–247.
16 Tafuri A, Alferink J, Moller P, Hammerling GJ, Arnold B: T cell awareness of paternal alloantigens during pregnancy. Science 1995;270:630–633.
17 Mellor AL, Sivakumar J, Chandler P, Smith K, Molina H, Mao D, Munn DH: Prevention of T cell-driven complement activation and inflammation by tryptophan catabolism during pregnancy. Nat Immunol 2001;2:64–68.
18 Heyborne K, Fu YX, Nelson A, Farr A, O'Brien R, Born W: Recognition of trophoblasts by γδ T cells. J Immunol 1994;153:2818–2976.
19 Wesch D, Glatzel A, Kabelitz D: Differentiation of resting human peripheral blood γδ T cells towards Th1- or Th2-phenotype. Cell Immunol 2001;212:110–117.
20 Clark DA, Flanders KC, Hirte H, Dasch JR, Coker R, McAnulty RJ, Laurent GJ: Characterization of murine pregnancy decidua TGF-β. I. TGFβ2-like molecules of unusual molecular size released in bioactive form. Biol Reprod 1995;52:1380–1388.
21 Lea RG, Underwood J, Flanders KC, Hirte H, Banwatt D, Finotto S, Ohno I, Daya S, Harley C, Michel M, Mowbray JF, Clark DA: A subset of patients with recurrent spontaneous abortion is deficient in transforming growth factor β2 producing 'suppressor cells' in uterine tissue near the placental attachment site. Am J Reprod Immunol 1995;34:52–63.
22 Clark DA, Arck PC, Chaouat G: Why did your mother reject you? Immunogenetic determinants of the response to environmental selective pressure expressed at the uterine level. Am J Reprod Immunol 1999;41:5–22.
23 Clark DA, Croitoru K: TH1/TH2 imbalance due to cytokine-producing NK, γδT and NKγδT cells in murine pregnancy decidua in success or failure of pregnancy. Am J Reprod Immunol 2001; 45:257–265.
24 Clark DA: Hard science versus phenomenology in reproductive immunology. Crit Rev Immunol 1999;19:509–539.
25 Potts WK, Manning CJ, Wakeland EK: Mating patterns in seminatural populations of mice influenced by MHC genotype. Nature 1991;352:619–621.
26 Chaouat, G, Clark DA, Wegmann TG: Genetic aspects of the CBA × DBA/2 and B10 × B10.A models of murine pregnancy failure and its prevention by lymphocyte immunization; in Beard RW,

Sharp F (eds): Early Pregnancy Loss: Mechanisms and Treatment. Ashton-under-Lyne, RCOG Peacock Press, 1988, pp 89–104.
27 Gorczynski RM, Chen Z, Kai Y, Lee L, Wong S, Marsden P: CD200 is a ligand for all members of the CD200 family of immunoregulatory molecules. J Immunol 2004;172:7744–7749.
28 Gorczynski RM, Chen Z, Clark DA, Kai Y, Lee L, Nachman J, Wong S, Marsden P: Structural and functional heterogeneity in the CD200R family of immunoregulatory molecules and their expression at the feto-maternal interface. Am J Reprod Immunol 2004;52:147–163.
29 Clark DA, Ding J, Yu G, Levy GA, Gorczynski R: Fgl2 prothrombinase expression in mouse trophoblast and decidua triggers abortion but may be countered by OX-2. Mol Hum Reprod 2001; 7:185–194.
30 Arck PC, Ferrick DA, Steele-Norwood D, Croitoru K, Clark DA: Murine T cell determination of pregnancy outcome. I. Effects of strain, αβ T cell receptor, γδ T cell receptor, and γδ T cell subsets. Am J Reprod Immunol 1997;37:492–502.
31 Clark DA, Chaouat G, Mogil R, Wegmann TG: Prevention of spontaneous abortion in DBA/2-mated CBA/J mice by GM-CSF involves CD8+ T cell-dependent suppression of natural effector cell cytotoxicity against trophoblast target cells. Cell Immunol 1994;154:143–152.
32 Clark DA, Chaouat G, Gorczynski RM: Thinking outside the box: Mechanisms of environmental selective pressure on the outcome of the materno-fetal relationship. Am J Reprod Immunol 2002; 47:275–282.
33 Aydintug MK, Roark CL, Yin X, Wands JM, Born WK, O'Brien RL: Detection of cell surface ligands for the γδ TCR using soluble TCRs. J Immunol 2004;172:4167–4175.
34 Zenclussen AC, Gerlof K, Zenclussen ML, Sollwedel A, Bertoja AZ, Ritter T, Kotsch K, Leber J, Volk HD: Abnormal T-cell reactivity against paternal antigens in spontaneous abortion: adoptive transfer of pregnancy-induced CD4+CD25+ T regulatory cells prevents fetal rejection in a murine abortion model. Am J Pathol 2005;166:811–822.
35 Aluvihare VR, Kallikourdis M, Betz AG: Regulatory T cells mediate maternal tolerance to the fetus. Nat Immunol 2004;5:266–271.
36 Gorczynski RM, Haddidi S, Yu G, Clark DA: The same immunoregulatory molecules contribute to successful pregnancy and transplantation. Am J Reprod Immunol 2002;48:18–26.
37 Clark DA, Yu G, Arck PC, Levy GA, Gorczynski RM: MD-1 is a critical part of the mechanism causing Th-1 cytokine-triggered murine fetal loss syndrome. Am J Reprod Immunol 2003; 49:297–307.
38 Desoye G, Dohr GA, Motter W, Winter R, Urdl W, Pusch H, Uchanska-Ziegler B, Zeigler A: Lack of HLA class I and class II antigens on human preimplantation embryos. J Immunol 1988; 140:4157–4159.
39 Hedley ML, Drake BL, Head JR, Tucker PW, Forman J: Differential expression of the class I MHC genes in the embryo and placenta during midgestational development in the mouse. J Immunol 1989;142:4046–4053.
40 Proll J, Blaschitz A, Hutter H, Dohr G: First trimester endovascular trophoblast cells express both HLA-C and HLA-G. Am J Reprod Immunol 1999;42:30–36.
41 Comiskey M, Goldstein CY, De Fazio SR, Mammolenti M, Newmark JA, Warner CM: Evidence that HLA-G is the functional analog of mouse Qa-2, the Ped gene product. Hum Immunol 2003; 64:999–1004.
42 Sipes SL, Medaglia MV, Stabley DL, DeBruyn CS, Alden MS, Catenacci V, Landel CP: A new histocompatibility complex class I b gene expressed in the mouse blastocyst and placenta. Immunogenetics 1996;45:108–120.
43 King A, Allan DS, Bowen M, Powis AJ, Joseph S, Verma S, Hiby SE, McMichael AJ, Loke YW, Braud VM: HLA-E is expressed on trophoblast and interacts with CD94/NKG2 receptors on decidual NK cells. Eur J Immunol 2000;30:1623–1631.
44 Le Bouteiller P: Major breakthrough in the HLA-G debate: Occurrence of pregnancy in humans depends on the HLA-G status of preimplantation embryos. Eur J Immunol 2002;32:309–310.
45 Ober C, Aldrich CL, Chervoneva I, Billstrand C, Rahimov F, Gray HL, Hyslop T: Variation in the HLA-G promoter region influences miscarriage rates. Am J Hum Genet 2003;72:1425–1435.

46 Chaouat G, Assal-Meliani A, Martal J, Raghupathy R, Elliot J, Mosmann T, Wegmann TG: IL-10 prevents naturally occurring fetal loss in the CBA × DBA/2 mating combination and local defect in IL-10 production in this abortion-prone combination is corrected by in vivo injection of IFN-τ. J Immunol 1995;154:4261–4268.
47 Kinsky R, Menu E, Chaouat G, Kapovic M, Jaulin C, Kourilsky P, Wegmann TG, Thang MN: The role of defined major histocompatibility antigens in preventing fetal death; in Chaouat G (ed): Immunology of Pregnancy. Boca Raton, CRC Press, 1993, pp 47–69.
48 Stallmach T, Arck P, Kagi D, Rulicke T: Pregnancy and perforin: What could be the role of a 'natural killer' in the decidua? Trophoblast Res 1998;12:143–150.
49 Reiger L, Hofmeister V, Probe C, Dietl J, Weiss EH, Steck T, Kammerer U: Th1- and Th2-like cytokine production by first trimester decidual large granular lymphocytes is influenced by HLA-G and HLA-E. Mol Hum Reprod 2002;8:255–261.
50 Rouas-Freiss N, LeMaoult J, Moreau P, Dausset J, Carosella ED: HLA-G in transplantation: A relevant molecule for inhibition of graft rejection? Am J Transplant 2003;3:11–16.
51 Hunt JS, Vasmer D, Ferguson TA, Miller L: FAS ligand is positioned in mouse uterus and placenta to prevent trafficking of activated leukocytes between mother and the conceptus. J Immunol 1997; 158:4122–4128.
52 Rogers AM, Boime I, Connolly J, Crook JR, Russell JH: Maternal-fetal tolerance is maintained despite transgene-driven trophoblast expression of MHC class I, and defects in FAS and its ligand. Eur J Immunol 1998;28:3479–3487.
53 Chaouat G, Clark DA: Fas/Fas ligand interaction at the placental interface is not required for the success of allogeneic pregnancy in anti-paternal MHC preimmunized mice. Am J Reprod Immunol 2001;45:108–115.
54 Munn DH, Zhou M, Attwood JT, Bonbdarev I, Conway SJ, Marshall B, Brown C, Mellor AL: Prevention of allogeneic fetal rejection by tryptophan catabolism. Science 1998;281:1191–1193.
55 Ito K, Karasawa M, Kawano T, Akasaka T, Koseki H, Akutsu Y, Kondo E, Sekiya S, Sekikawa K, Harada M, Yamashita M, Nakayama T, Taniguchi M: Involvement of decidua Vα14 NKT cells in abortion. Proc Natl Acad Sci USA 2000;97:740–744.
56 Clark DA, Blois S, Kandil J, Handjiski B, Manuel J, Arck PC: Reduced indoleamine 2,3-diokygenous versus increased Th1/Th2 cytokine ratios as a basis for occult and clinical pregnancy failure in mice and humans. Submitted for publication.
57 Kinsky R, Delage G, Rosin N, Thang MN, Hoffman M, Chaouat G: A murine model of NK cell mediated resorption. Am J Reprod Immunol 1990;23:73–77.

Professor David A. Clark, MD, PhD, FRCP(C), FRCP
McMaster University, 1200 Main St. West Rm 3V39
Hamilton, Ont. L8N 3Z5 (Canada), Tel. +1 905 521 2100, ext. 76376
Fax +1 905 521 4971, E-Mail clarkd@mcmaster.ca

Markert UR (ed): Immunology of Pregnancy.
Chem Immunol Allergy. Basel, Karger, 2005, vol 89, pp 49–61

Immunology of Preeclampsia

Leif Matthiesen[a], Göran Berg[a], Jan Ernerudh[b], Christina Ekerfelt[b], Yvonne Jonsson[b], Surendra Sharma[c]

[a]Department of Molecular and Clinical Medicine, Division of Obstetrics and Gynaecology and [b]Department of Molecular and Clinical Medicine, Division of Clinical Immunology, University Hospital, Linkoping, Sweden; [c]Department of Pediatrics and Pathology, Women and Infants Hospital of Rhode Island, Brown University, Providence, R.I., USA

Abstract

Preeclampsia is a placenta-dependent disorder with both local and systemic anomalies with neonatal and maternal morbidity. It is manifested late in pregnancy, but the onset is during early stages of gestation. The current hypothesis regarding the aetiology of preeclampsia is focused on maladaptation of immune responses and defective trophoblast invasion. Thus, an excessive maternal inflammatory response, perhaps directed against foreign fetal antigens, results in a chain of events including shallow trophoblast invasion, defective spiral artery remodelling, placental infarction and release of pro-inflammatory cytokines and placental fragments in the systemic circulation. During normal pregnancy, trophoblasts interact in the decidua with the unique uterine NK cells, modifying their cytokine repertoire, regulating adhesion molecules and matrix metalloproteinases. The inability of trophoblasts to accomplish these changes might be a critical factor for the onset of preeclampsia. Several cytokines, produced at the maternal-fetal interface, have an impact on trophoblast invasion. It is suggested that deficiency of interleukin-10 may contribute to enhanced inflammatory responses towards the trophoblasts elicited by e.g. tumour necrosis factor-α and interferon-γ. Consequently, trophoblasts subjected to a high rate of apoptosis are hampered in their invasive capacity resulting in defective transformation of spiral arteries, hypoxia, thrombosis and infarction of the placenta. The ensuing infarction of placenta leads to leakage of increasing amounts of placental fragments and cytokines in the maternal circulation and an exaggerated systemic endothelial activation as identified in preeclampsia. So far, treatment of preeclampsia is focused on signs like hypertension, whereas attempts of modifying immune responses may be a possibility in the future.

Introduction

Preeclampsia is a complication that is detected in the second half of pregnancy, but most probably has its onset during the early stages of gestation. This pregnancy-associated disorder is histologically characterized by restrained trophoblast invasion, vasculitis, thrombosis and ischaemia of the placenta. These features may also be apparent in other obstetric complications like recurrent spontaneous abortion, intrauterine growth retardation, fetal death, and abruptio placentae. The seemingly disparate clinical entities might have their common aetiology in the immune responses including local subclinical inflammation at the placental bed and systemically (in preeclampsia) in the maternal circulation. Preeclampsia is hard to detect in its early form and predictors that can be used to identify the women at risk of preeclampsia would be of value for the clinician. This paper deals with preeclampsia in humans and associated immunological changes and is an overview of recent important findings of this important but still poorly understood condition.

Clinical Preeclampsia

Preeclampsia occurs after the 20th week of gestation and is a heterogeneous disease. Since termination of pregnancy cures the disease, preeclampsia is a placenta-dependent disorder with both local intrauterine and systemic signs and symptoms. The hallmark signs are hypertension and proteinuria (table 1). The incidence of preeclampsia is 3–5% of all pregnancies depending on the population studied [1].

A number of risk factors are thought to increase the risk of developing preeclampsia: maternal vascular disease, autoimmune disorders, maternal and paternal genetic causes, diabetes mellitus, primiparity and twin pregnancy. Although the exact aetiology remains to be delineated, all of the associated causes converge into a common pathophysiological denominator: endothelial dysfunction. Thus, it has been suggested that an excessive maternal inflammatory response, perhaps directed against foreign fetal antigens, results in an impaired trophoblast invasion with a defective spiral artery remodelling ensued by high-resistance vessels and a reduced placental perfusion. The consequences are placental hypoxia and infarction with release of pro-inflammatory cytokines and placental fragments into the maternal circulation with ultimately generalized maternal, and possibly fetal, endothelial activation [1].

Trophoblast Invasion

An adequate trophoblast invasion is possible only after a proper endometrial decidualization of the uterine wall has occurred. The decidualization is initiated immediately after ovulation in order to receive the embryo. The production of progesterone from the corpus luteum stimulates the decidua to

Table 1. Diagnosis of preeclampsia

Definition of preeclampsia according to WHO
Preeclampsia is a syndrome defined by hypertension and proteinuria and may be associated with other signs and symptoms
Preeclampsia occurs after the 20th gestational week
Moderate preeclampsia
Systolic blood pressure ≥140 mm Hg and/or a diastolic pressure ≥90 mm Hg measured on separate occasions at least 4 h apart
Proteinuria in a 24-hour protein excretion ≥300 mg or 1+ on two random urine samples collected 4 h apart
Severe preeclampsia
Systolic blood pressure >160 mm Hg and/or diastolic ≥110 mm Hg measured on separate occasions at least 4 h apart
Proteinuria in a 24-hour protein excretion ≥5 g or 3+ on two random urine samples collected 4 h apart
Cerebral dysfunction (blurred vision, scotoma, headache, cerebrovascular accidents)
Epigastric or right upper quadrant pain
Renal failure or oliguria ≤500 ml in 24 h
Pulmonary oedema
Impaired liver function (serum transaminase levels 2 times normal or greater)
Thrombocytopenia (≤100,000 platelets/mm^3)
Coagulopathy
Fetal growth restriction
Eclampsia (generalized convulsions)
HELLP

increase the vascularization and secretory activity of the endometrial glands. The leukocytes in the decidua consist mainly of unique uterine natural killer (uNK) cells (65–70%) and monocyte/macrophages (15–20%), whose exact function is unknown. A small number of T cells are also present, whereas B cells are almost absent. In the endometrial extracellular matrix (consisting of different types of collagens, proteoglycans, and glycoproteins), changes occur facilitating the invasive properties of trophoblasts creating a safe anchor of the placenta in the decidua and the vascular remodelling of the spiral arteries [2, 3].

The invading cytotrophoblasts are a subpopulation of villous cytotrophoblasts, which in turn differentiate into an outer layer of multinucleated cells, the syncytiotrophoblasts. The syncytiotrophoblasts cover the fetal mesenchyme and blood vessels and are in direct contact with maternal circulating blood. Across this syncytiotrophoblast cell membrane, nutrients and oxygen are delivered to the fetus and waste products are returned to the maternal circulation.

The cytotrophoblasts that differentiate into extravillous cytotrophoblasts are designed to develop a migratory capacity to invade deep into the decidual matrix and the maternal spiral arteries. The musculoelastic media of the spiral arteries are replaced by the invading cytotrophoblasts and fibrinoid material. The spiral arteries are thereby modulated into low-resistance flow channels allowing increased blood volume to the intervillous space [3]. The invasion of cytotrophoblasts relies on their expression of cell adhesion molecules and secretion of proteolytic enzymes, matrix metalloproteinases (MMP). Integrins are cell membrane adhesion receptors that adhere to different matrix glycoproteins depending on their expression of tissue-specific αβ subunits. When trophoblasts migrate across the basement membrane and into the decidua towards the spiral arteries their expression of integrins is modulated according to the structure of the surrounding tissue. The surrounding matrix is digested by proteolytic enzymes secreted by the trophoblasts. Thus, the integrins and proteases together give trophoblasts a migratory capacity, which is a significant physiological adaptation for a successful pregnancy outcome. A shallow trophoblast invasion results in a poor placenta vascularization and deficient anchor in the matrix tissue. This is associated with a high risk of preeclampsia, intrauterine growth retardation and abruptio placentae [3–5].

Balancing Act between Inflammatory and Anti-Inflammatory Immune Responses

The trophoblast invasion is under the influence of several cytokines produced at the maternal-fetal interface by several cells of immune and non-immune origin, such as leucocytes including NK cells, trophoblasts, stromal cells and glandular endothelium [6]. Thus, the current hypothesis regarding the aetiology of preeclampsia should focus on maladaptation of immune responses and defective trophoblast invasion (fig. 1). The activation of the adaptive immune response is characterized according to the phenomenon of polarized cytokine secretion by T helper (Th) cells. These are primarily divided into two subsets: Th1 and Th2. In humans, Th1 cells secrete inflammatory cytokines such as interferon-γ (IFNI-γ) and tumour necrosis factor-α (TNF-α), whereas Th2 cells secrete anti-inflammatory cytokines such as IL-4, IL-5, and IL-9. Both Th1 and Th2 cells as well as non-lymphoid cells, including macrophages, secrete IL-10. Although the Th1/Th2 model is too simple to encompass all the complex differentiation profiles of cytokine-producing cells, it still provides a useful framework to explain the immune responses imparted either by immune cells or non-immune cells [7].

An important decisive factor for the induction of either the Th1 or Th2 pathway is the presence of certain cytokines during the initial process when

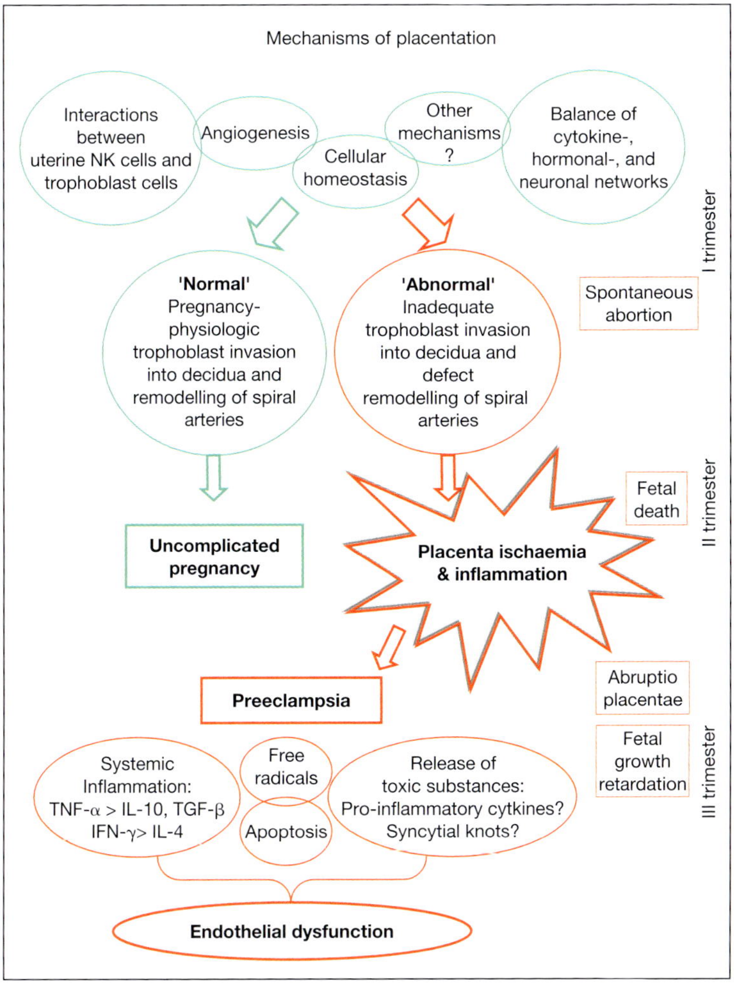

Fig. 1. Flow chart showing mechanisms of placental development in uncomplicated pregnancies ('normal') and of pathological placentation ('abnormal'), as in preeclampsia. Other pregnancy complications, spontaneous abortion, fetal death and growth retardation, may also be clinical signs of placental ischaemia and inflammation as shown.

antigens are recognized. IL-4 dictates the immune response to Th2 and the effects of IL-4 have been shown to dominate over those of IFN-γ [8]. Thus, it is possible that the presence of the trophoblasts in a uterine cavity with a poor resident anti-inflammatory milieu initiates an incompatible activation of the decidual immune cells that direct the local immune activity towards inflammation.

Subsequently, the systemic cytokine production and immune responses are likely to be predominant in their inflammatory functions which might initiate the pathology associated with preeclampsia.

Cytokines and Preeclampsia

A set of cytokines have so far been of particular interest in the pathological pregnancy outcome, including preeclampsia (fig. 1).

Transforming Growth Factor-β

Transforming growth factor-β (TGF-β) is secreted by decidual stroma cells, macrophages and T cells and is present locally at the maternal-fetal interface. This cytokine exerts a regulatory role by a potent negative effect on trophoblast invasiveness by induction of tissue inhibitors of matrix proteases and increased adhesiveness to matrix proteins [5, 6]. However, the impact of an overexpression of TGF-β on a shallow cytotrophoblast invasion at the fetal-placental unit has been disputed since no difference was found either in the placental bed or in the placenta in preeclamptic patients compared with normal pregnancies [9].

Tumour Necrosis Factor-α

TNF-α is a proinflammatory cytokine produced e.g. by NK cells, monocytes/macrophages and trophoblasts. TNF-α promotes apoptosis and leakage of the endothelial vessels, leading to systemic endothelial activation and thereby signs associated with preelampsia [10]. In conjunction with an overexpression and secretion of TNF-α in the placenta and in plasma – as observed in preeclampsia – an enhanced plasma and placental expression of IL-1 has been reported. IL-1 and TNF-α both promote structural and functional changes in endothelial cells including oxidative stress, activation of the complement cascade, secretion of vasoconstrictors, microthrombosis and infarction, and elevated thromboxane levels. All these changes are seen in preeclampsia and the effects of increased expression of TNF-α seem to be involved in the pathophysiological mechanisms leading to the clinical signs [1, 11]. Thus, TNF-α is a major contributor to many of the local and systemic changes that characterize preeclampsia. TNF-α has also been shown to elevate leptin protein levels, a phenomenon associated with preeclampsia. Interestingly, microarray analysis of differentially expressed genes in placental tissue of preeclampsia revealed that one of the most upregulated transcripts in preeclampsia tissue was the obese leptin gene [12].

Interferon-γ

IFN-γ released by activated T cells activates the specialized uNK cells which possess regulatory properties for physiological trophoblast invasion in the decidua. However, excessive amounts of IFN-γ in conjunction with TNF-α and IL-1 can lead to apoptosis of trophoblasts [2, 13]. This may indeed also be the case in unexplained spontaneous abortions [14]. In an inflammatory environment, macrophages secrete high levels of IL-12 that stimulate IFN-γ secretion by NK cells, thereby inhibiting angiogenesis [6].

IL-10

IL-10 is an important anti-inflammatory cytokine in pregnancy that inhibits upregulation of MMP-2 and MMP-9 and promotes the termination of Th1 inflammatory rejection reactions against the fetal-placental unit. In a small number of preeclampsia cases, high levels of IL-10 are seen both in the placenta and in peripheral blood, which might be a compensatory response to elevated levels of IFN-γ, TNF-α, IL-2 and IL-12 [5, 8, 15]. On the other hand, IL-10 deficiency and an increase of TNF-α expression in the placenta and decidua are observed in preeclampsia compared to those with a normal pregnancy. This was interpreted as a modified immune balance consistent with inflammatory responses in preeclampsia [16]. This suggests that coupling of IL-10 deficiency and inflammatory signals at different stages of pregnancy may contribute to disparate clinical conditions, including preeclampsia [17, Sharma, unpubl. observations].

Other Cytokines

Recently, several other cytokines have been identified in the immunopathological cascade of preeclampsia. Since these cytokines do not adjust to the original concept of Th2 as beneficial and Th1 as deleterious to pregnancy, it has been proposed that caution should be observed with the immunotrophism theory stated by Wegmann et al. [18]. Nevertheless, the Th1/Th2 paradigm in its simplistic form may still be part of complex immune-endocrine interactions locally or systemically. In this context, Chaouat et al. [19] suggest that the preclinical cytokine network has come closer to the patient bedside, showing a correlation between the evaluation of uterine blood flow, ultrasonographic morphology of uterine-placental vessels and immunohistochemical localization and levels of IL-12, IL-18 and counts of uNK cells. They showed, in a group of patients enrolled in an in vitro fertilization programme, that a correlation exists between cytotoxic cytokine profiles and vascular anomalies in implantation failures. This scenario is in contrast with the proper activation and localization of uNK cells and vasculature seen in implantation success. Pro-inflammatory cytokines trigger activation of the coagulation cascade leading to vasculitis and infarction and may further deteriorate the early placental development and hamper the trophoblast invasion [1, 5, 10].

Recently, an elegant way of measuring cytotoxic responses, by means of granulysin levels in serum, was reported to be associated with the occurrence and clinical manifestations of preeclampsia [20]. The real challenge is to find early markers of subsequent preeclampsia. In this context, soluble IL-2 receptor in plasma was elevated in the 1st trimester of women that later developed preeclampsia compared with controls [21].

Maternal-Fetal Interactions

In the uterine cavity, the extravillous cytotrophoblast cells reveal themselves by the expression of the unusual HLA class I molecules: HLA-E, and HLA-G together with HLA-C. At present, the only receptors that have been found to these HLA class I molecules are located on the unique uNK cells (fig. 1). uNK cells are CD56bright CD16– compatible with a low cytotoxic potential compared with the classical killer NK cells in peripheral blood that express CD56dim CD16+. The syncytiotrophoblast, covering the placental villi and thereby exposed to maternal blood, expresses no HLA molecules [2].

The uNK cells show a variation over the menstrual period. During the luteal phase and until midgestation uNK cells increase in number and they accumulate around the invading cytotrophoblasts. After initial development of the placenta, levels of uNK cells decline and cease to be present at term [2].

The interaction between extravillous cytotrophoblasts and uNK cells, possibly after stimulation by IFN-γ, has recently been suggested to have an influence on the remodelling of spiral arteries [22]. A high expression of receptors signalling inhibition of cytotoxic activity of uNK cells interacts with HLA-E, HLA-C, and HLA-G [2].

The inability of cytotrophoblasts to modify the cytokine repertoire of uNK cells and their regulation of adhesion molecules, MMPs and sufficient neovascularization may be critical factors for the onset of pregnancy complications including preeclampsia [2, 3, 6, 17, 18].

Apoptosis and Syncytial Knots

Programmed cell death or apoptosis plays an important role in cell homeostasis and tissue remodelling, particularly placental development. Importantly, placental degeneration observed in preeclampsia may be due to unscheduled apoptosis of trophoblasts. The pregnancy-associated remodelling of the spiral arteries is mediated by invasive cytotrophoblasts. However, if these trophoblasts are subjected to a high rate of apoptosis, this defective transformation of spiral arteries may result in local ischaemia, thrombosis and infarction (fig. 1). The exact causes of enhanced apoptosis in preeclampsia are currently unknown. Likewise, increased apoptosis of syncytiotrophoblasts may increase the amount of syncytiotrophoblast debris, syncytial knots, that leak into the maternal circulation and generate an exaggerated systemic endothelial activation [23]. Sargent et al. [24] have proposed that when syncytial knots break off in increasing amounts from the placenta and are shed into the maternal circulation they may be the cause of the systemic endothelial activation that is seen in preeclampsia (fig. 1). The deported trophoblast debris can, in vitro, activate maternal sources of TNF-α and IL-12 from monocytes, which further pushes the systemic immune response towards extensive inflammation instead of the normal innate immune reactivity that syncytial knots usually accomplish during pregnancy. The reason for this strong apoptosis is unknown, but it has been shown that pro-inflammatory cytokines are capable of upregulating Fas/FasL genes, while anti-inflammatory cytokines protect trophoblasts against Fas-induced apoptosis [24, Sharma, unpubl. observations].

Free Radicals

Other mediators of inflammation are also important in the pathogenesis of preeclampsia, including reactive oxygen species, in particular superoxide anions. These agents are increased in preeclampsia, where the equilibrium of antioxidants (vitamin E, ascorbic acid, glutathione peroxidase, superoxide catalase/mutase, and caeruloplasmin) is disturbed. Antioxidants are produced by many cells, also trophoblasts and leucocytes, to protect them from free radicals or as part of cellular homeostasis and ageing. Free radicals and levels of lipid peroxidation are increased in preeclampsia and capable of evoking systemic endothelial activation, including platelet consumption, altered thromboxane/prostacyclin ratio, increased TNF-α production and promotion of the coagulation cascade [25].

During normal pregnancy, a rise in antioxidants is detected in blood with increasing gestational age. However, if the inflammation is strong or the production of the antioxidants is low, the predominating condition inevitably favours oxidizing species. This is the case in preeclampsia, where free radicals are present at significantly higher levels than during normal pregnancy [25] (fig. 1). In the 'haemolysis, elevated liver enzymes, low platelet' (HELLP) syndrome, haemolysis of erythrocytes might occur due to a high degree of oxidation of glutathione, which causes cell damage. As a consequence, it has been suggested that treatment with inhibitors of cyclooxygenase to block oxidative stress on erythrocytes as well as nutritional supplements with antioxidants, vitamin E and C, might reduce the incidence of preeclampsia in high-risk pregnancies [25].

Lymphocyte Populations in Blood

Preeclampsia is also characterized by systemic changes in the distribution of lymphocyte populations in peripheral blood. Increased levels of activated/memory cells (CD4+CD45RO+ and CD4+CD29+) and decreased levels of naïve/'suppressor' cells (CD4+CD45RA+) have been noted. The interpretation is that antigens have activated the T cells observed in preeclampsia. In contrast, lymphocytes in normal pregnancy are switched towards a predominance of CD4+CD45RA+ naïve/'suppressor' T cells. The level of cytotoxic CD8+ T cells expressing the S6F1 marker, which represent killer effector functions, is increased in preeclamptic pregnancies compared with normal pregnancies, again indicating inflammatory activity [26].

The mechanisms behind leucocyte activation in preeclampsia are unknown, but the changes are similar to those observed in humans after viral or bacterial infections. Low doses of bacterial endotoxin injected into pregnant rats resulted in a condition resembling preeclampsia including the appearance of T cell activation markers [15]. This presents an intriguing basis to probe the role of clinical and subclinical infections in the pathogenesis of preeclampsia. These observations also indicate that preeclampsia is associated with both the innate and the adaptive immune activity in the peripheral blood [6, 18, 24, 26].

Toxic Substances of Preeclampsia

What is the nature of the 'toxic' substances that escape from an obvious 'sick' placenta, swim out into the maternal circulation and gain access to and disturb almost every organ in the human body and reveal their presence by the characteristic signs and symptoms of preeclampsia (fig. 1)? Many candidates (fig. 1) have been suggested although no complete agreement has been reached [1, 6, 10, 11, 16, 18, 23–25].

Concerning cytokines as potential villains and as potential diagnostic tools in the prediction of preeclampsia, we addressed this question (like many others) by measuring cytokine levels in serum using the Luminex® assay (Camarillo, Calif., USA) in preeclamptic patients (n = 15) and compared them with normal pregnancies (n = 15). In preeclampsia, we observed an upregulated systemic innate immune reactivity with increased levels of TNF-α, IL-6, and IL-8. When we stimulated peripheral blood mononuclear cells with paternal antigens ('fetus-specific') or recall antigens (purified protein derivates of *Mycobacterium tuberculosis* or tetanus toxoid) similar levels of induced secretions of IL-4, IL-10, IL-12 and IFN-γ (detected by the highly sensitive ELISPOT assay) were detected in preeclampsia and normal pregnancies. This does not exclude local cytokine aberrations at the placental level that are compatible with inflammatory activity. However, the results agree with the main concept of preeclampsia being an inflammatory phenomenon [1, 6, 15, 18, 23, 24], but with a much more complex picture than a Th1 deviation only [19].

Conclusion

Preeclampsia is a multisystem disorder based on a cascade of immunopathological events originating from the placenta. No single candidate mechanism exists to explain the complex pathogenesis. As of now, there is no reliable marker or predictor of preeclampsia. Clearly, however, local as well as systemic inflammatory activity occurs in preeclamptic patients. To identify these complex immune factors and 'arrange' them in a test where the diverted inflammatory activity will be detected should be the target in future research concerning preeclampsia.

To further elucidate the mechanisms underlying preeclampsia, it is our hope that animal models can be developed in the very near future, wherein depletion or the overwhelming presence of key players in the aetiology of the disease can be studied developmentally.

Acknowledgment

This study was supported by the US Public Health COBRE grant 1 P20 RR018728 (SS) NIH, a grant of the County Council of Östergötland, Sweden and a grant of the Health Research Council in the South-East of Sweden.

References

1 Roberts JM, Taylor RN, Musci TJ, Rodgers GM, Hubel CA, McLaughlin MK: Preeclampsia: An endothelial cell disorder. Am J Obstet Gynecol 1999;54:133–142.

2 Moffett-King A: Natural killer cells and pregnancy. Nat Rev Immunol 2002;2:656–663.

3 Bischof P, Campana A: A model for implantation of the human blastocyst and early placentation. Hum Reprod Update 1996; 2/3:262–270.
4 Pijnenborg R: The placental bed. Hypertens Pregnancy 1996;15:7–23.
5 Zhou Y, Fisher SJ, Janatpour M, Genbacev O, Dejana E, Wheelock M, Damsky CH: Human cytotrophoblast adopt a vascular phenotype as they differentiate. A strategy for successful endovascular invasion? J Clin Invest 1997;99:2139–2151.
6 Saito S, Sakai M: Th1/Th2 balance in preeclampsia. J Reprod Immunol 2003;59:161–173.
7 Mosmann TR, Sad S: The expanding universe of T-cell subsets: Th1, Th2 and more. Immunol Today 1996;17:138–146.
8 Swain SL: IL-4 dictates T-cell differentiation. Res Immunol 1993;144:616–620.
9 Lyall F, Simpson H, Bulmer JN, Barber A, Robson SC: Transforming growth factor-β expression in human placenta and placental bed in third trimester normal pregnancy, preeclampsia, and fetal growth restriction. Am J Pathol 2001;159:1827–1838.
10 Rinehart BK, Terrone DA, Lagoo-Deenadayalan S, Barber WH, Hale EA, Martin JN, Bennett WA: Expression of the placental cytokines tumor necrosis factor α, interleukin 1β and interleukin 10 is increased in preeclampsia. Am J Obstet Gynecol 1999;181:915–920.
11 Anim-Nyame N, Gamble J, Sooranna SR, Johnson MR, Steer PJ: Microvascular permeability is related to circulating levels of tumour necrosis factor-α in pre-eclampsia. Cardiovasc Res 2003; 58:162–169.
12 Reimer T, Koczan D, Gerber B, Richter D, Theisen HJ, Friese K: Microarray analysis of differentially expressed genes in placental tissue of pre-eclampsia: Up-regulation of obesity related genes. Mol Hum Reprod 2002;8:674–680.
13 Ashkar AA, DiSanto JP, Croy BA: Interferon-gamma contributes to initiation of uterine vascular modification, decidual integrity, and uterine natural killer cell maturation during normal murine pregnancy. J Exp Med 2000;192:259–270.
14 Plevyak M, Hanna N, Mayer S, Murphy S, Pinar H, Fast L, Ekerfelt C, Ernerudh J, Berg G, Matthiesen L, Sharma S: Deficiency of decidual IL-10 in first trimester missed abortion: A lack of correlation with the decidual immune cell profile. Am J Reprod Immunol 2002;47: 242–250.
15 Murphy S, Fast L, Sharma S: IL-10, uterine NK cells, inflammation, and pregnancy. Am J Reprod Immunol 2004;51:434.
16 Henessy A, Pilmore HL, Simmons LA, Painter DM: A deficiency of placental IL-10 in preeclampsia. J Immunol 1999;163:3491–3495.
17 Roth I, Fisher SJ: IL-10 is an autocrine inhibitor of human placental cytotrophoblast MMP-9 production and invasion. Dev Biol 1999;205:194–204.
18 Wegmann TG, Lin H, Guilbert L, Mossman TH: Bidirectional cytokine interactions in the materno-fetal relationship: Is successful pregnancy a Th2 phenomenon? Immunol Today 1993; 14:353–355.
19 Chaouat G, Ledee-Bataille N, Zourbas S, Dubanchat S, Sandra O, Martal J, Ostojojic S, Frydman R: Implantation: Can immunological parameters of implantation failure be of interest for preeclampsia? J Reprod Immunol 2003;59:205–217.
20 Sakai M, Ogawa K, Shiozaki A, Yoneda S, Sasaki Y, Nagata K, Saito S: Serum granulysin is a marker for Th1 type immunity in pre-eclampsia. Clin Exp Immunol 2004;1:114–119.
21 Eneroth E, Remberger M, Vahlne A, Ringden O: Increased serum concentrations of interleukin-2 receptor in the first trimester in women who later developed severe preeclampsia. Acta Obstet Gynecol Scand 1998;77:591–593.
22 Croy BA, Ashkar AA, Minhas K, Greenwood JD: Can murine uterine natural killer cells give insights into the pathogenesis of pre eclampsia? J Soc Gynecol Invest 2000;7:12–20.
23 Neale D, Demasio K, Illuzi J, Chaiworapongsa T, Romero R, Mor G: Maternal serum of women with pre-eclampsia reduces trophoblast cell viability: Evidence for an increased sensitivity to Fas-mediated apoptosis. J Maternal Fetal Neonatal Med 2003;13:39–44.
24 Sargent IL, Germain SJ, Sacks GP, Kumar S, Redman CWG: Trophoblast deportation and the maternal inflammatory response in pre-eclampsia. J Reprod Immunol 2003;59:153–160.

25 Walker JJ: Antioxidants and inflammatory cell responses in preeclampsia. Semin Reprod Endocrinol 1998;16/1:47–55.
26 Matthiesen L, Berg G, Ernerudh J, Skogh T: Lymphocyte subsets and autoantibodies in pregnancies complicated by placental disorders. Am J Reprod Immunol 1995;33:31–39.
27 Jonsson Y, Rubèr M, Matthiesen L, Berg G. Nieminen K, Sharma S, Ernerudh J, Ekerfelt C: Cytokine mapping of serum from women with preeclampsia and from women with normal pregnancy. Am J Reprod Immunol, submitted.

Leif Matthiesen
Department of Molecular and Clinical Medicine
Division of Obstetrics and Gynaecology, University Hospital
SE–581 85 Linkoping (Sweden), Tel. +46 13 22 31 37
Fax +46 13 14 81 56, E-Mail leif.matthiesen@lio.se

Markert UR (ed): Immunology of Pregnancy.
Chem Immunol Allergy. Basel, Karger, 2005, vol 89, pp 62–71

TNF-α-Mediated Stress-Induced Early Pregnancy Loss: A Possible Role of Leukemia Inhibitory Factor

A. Torchinsky[a], *U.R. Markert*[b], *V. Toder*[a]

[a]Department of Cell and Developmental Biology, Sackler School of Medicine, Tel Aviv University, Tel Aviv, Israel; [b]Placenta-Labor, Abteilung für Geburtshilfe, Friedrich-Shiller-Universität, Jena, Germany

Abstract

Background: Leukemia inhibitory factor (LIF) is at present suggested to be essential for implantation in mammals. In parallel, the possibility that it may also be involved in the pathogenesis of stress-induced early embryonic death seems to emerge from studies, which addressed the embryotoxic potential of another cytokine, tumor necrosis factor-α (TNF-α). In this brief review, we discuss this possibility based on these studies as well as on those addressing TNF-α and LIF signaling. **Methods:** Existing data were reviewed critically. **Results:** Data summarized in this review suggest that: (1) TNF-α may act as a mediator of stress-induced early embryonic death, (2) TNF-α-mediated early embryonic death induced by some detrimental stimuli may be attributed to a dysfunction of mechanisms, which are critical for the ability of the uterus to become receptive to blastocysts, allowing implantation, (3) one such mechanism was shown to be associated with LIF signaling in uterine cells, and (4) TNF-α seems to have the potential to affect LIF signaling. **Conclusion:** Data presented in the this review suggest LIF as a good candidate for further studies addressing molecular mechanisms underlying stress-induced early embryonic death.

Introduction

Early embryonic death is the main adverse result of various harmful maternal stimuli or environmental embryopathic stresses acting before or during implantation [1]. Studies addressing the pathogenesis of this phenomenon revealed that stresses inducing embryonic death also alter the production of some cytokines operating in the embryonic microenvironment [2, 3]. As the balance between various cytokines acting in the embryonic vicinity was shown to be an essential condition for a successful pregnancy [4], these observations suggested a role for cytokines as regulators of the embryo's response to embryotoxic stimuli.

Leukemia inhibitory factor (LIF), a proinflammatory cytokine, was shown to be essential for implantation in mice [5]. Maybe, due to this fact, its role in mediating stress-induced early embryonic death remains practically uninvestigated. At the same time, such a role seems to emerge from studies which addressed the embryotoxic potential of another cytokine, tumor necrosis factor-α (TNF-α). In this brief review, we summarize results of these studies and discuss whether LIF may be involved in the pathogenesis of TNF-α-mediated stress-induced early embryonic death. Since there is a plethora of reviews addressing the role of both cytokines in reproduction as well as TNF-α and LIF signaling, we will not address this topic here in detail but will focus only on points which have relevance to the topic of the review.

TNF-α as an Inducer of Embryonic Death

TNF-α, a multifunctional cytokine, was identified in the ovary, oviduct, uterus and placenta practically at all stages of development [6]. Although results of a number of studies suggested its functional role in reproduction (especially in implantation) [references in 6], experiments in TNF-α knockout mice [7, 8] revealed neither alterations in indices characterizing their reproductive performance nor structural anomalies in fetuses, indicating that the cytokine hardly plays an essential role in regulating the antenatal period of development. At the same time, there is a large body of data, which, taken together, suggest its involvement in mediating spontaneous and stress-induced early embryonic death [9]. These data may briefly be summarized as follows.

(1) The embryotoxic potential of the cytokine seems to have been suggested for the first time by studies demonstrating that injection of TNF-α into pregnant mice results in embryonic death [10]. Further experiments in the CBA/J × DBA/2J mouse combination (a model with a high incidence of embryonic death) have revealed an increased level of TNF-α in supernatants of decidual cell cultures [10]. TNF-α expression has also been found to be raised in the placentae of CBA/J × DBA/2J mice [11]. These observations have implicated TNF-α as a cytokine involved in triggering immunological pregnancy loss [12], i.e. death of embryos due to failure of defense mechanisms preventing rejection of the semiallogeneic fetoplacental unit.

(2) The ability of TNF-α to influence the preimplantation development of embryos seems to be well documented. Thus, rat blastocysts exposed to TNF-α exhibited decreased cell proliferation [13] and an increased rate of blastomere apoptosis [14]. Practically the same results have been observed in studies with cultured mouse and cattle blastocysts [15, 16]. Remarkably, the possibility that this impact of TNF-α on preimplantation embryos could be detrimental is clearly demonstrated by embryo transfer studies addressing in vivo development of blastocysts, which were exposed in vitro to TNF-α [15]. They revealed that TNF-α pretreatment caused a 17% decrease in the proportion of implanted embryos and that the proportion of embryos, which died after implantation, was about 40% higher in the TNF-α-pretreated group as compared to controls.

There are a number of studies which suggest that uterine cells may also serve as targets for the toxic effect of TNF-α. Thus, experiments in the mouse uterine epithelial cell line WEG-1 revealed that TNF-α exerts a dose- and time-dependent toxic effect on these cells while stimulating apoptosis [17]. The human endometrial HEC-1 cell line was found also to be sensitive to the toxic effect of the cytokine [18]. Finally, the possibility that TNF-α may be involved in pathological processes, leading to pregnancy loss by disturbing normal trophoblast endocrine function, has also been demonstrated [19].

(3) Three types of data exist suggesting an involvement of TNF-α in the pathogenesis of stress-induced early embryonic death.

First, data demonstrating that stress-induced cell death was accompanied by an upregulation of TNF-α expression in embryonic vicinity. Thus, elevated TNF-α expression has been observed in the uterine epithelium and stroma, and in the giant and spongiotrophoblast cells of the placenta of mice exposed to the DNA-damaging agent cyclophosphamide [20]. Increased production of TNF-α by decidual NK cells and/or macrophages has been observed in mice treated with LPS [21]. TNF-α-producing cells located at the fetomaternal interface have been observed to be activated and to increase the local production of TNF-α in mice exposed to ultrasonic sound stress [22]. Finally, studies in diabetic animals, which demonstrate a dramatic decrease in pregnancy rate [23], have revealed that the synthesis of TNF-α is upregulated in the uterine cells of these mice [18, 24].

Second, data demonstrating that maternal immunostimulation, which increased the resistance of embryos to various embryopathic stresses [3], also partially normalized (decreased) the expression of TNF-α at the fetomaternal interface. This phenomenon was observed in experiments with immunostimulated mice exposed to ultrasound stress, cyclophosphamide and LPS as well as in immunostimulated diabetic mice [references in 3].

Finally, the involvement of the cytokine in mediating stress-induced cell death is also suggested by studies in TNF-α knockout mice. Thus, TNF-α was shown to be essential to mediate embryonic death induced by α-galactosylceramide, a specific ligand for a distinct subset of lymphocytes, Va14 NKT cells, which accumulate in the decidua during pregnancy [25]. Also, in a study with diabetic mice [26] we observed a much greater decrease in the pregnancy rate in severely diabetic TNF-$\alpha^{+/+}$ mice than in TNF-$\alpha^{-/-}$ mice. The comparative analysis of results obtained in diabetic mice tested on days 4, 8 and 18 of pregnancy suggests that this decrease could be due to TNF-α-induced death of peri-implantation embryos.

The Blastocyst and Uterus as Targets for TNF-α

In vitro studies with blastocysts exposed to TNF-α revealed that the cytokine predominantly induces a deficit in fetal precursor cells situated in the inner cell mass but not in preplacental cells situated in the trophectoderm [references in 18]. These observations are in a good agreement with embryo transfer experiments, which demonstrated that TNF-α-pretreated blastocysts implanted at about the same rate as control embryos but the resorption rate (postimplantation death) was significantly higher among embryos exposed to the cytokine [15]. Together, these results suggest that TNF-α acting on blastocysts decreases mainly their ability to differentiate into fetuses after implantation rather than their ability to implant in the uterus.

Since TNF-α-treated blastocysts were transferred to intact females, the pattern of the embryonic death observed in these experiments reflects a situation, where only blastocysts but not females are exposed to the embryopathic stress. At the same time, the pattern of embryonic death demonstrated by diabetic females dramatically differed from that observed in the above-mentioned embryo transfer experiments.

As we mentioned the above, diabetes was shown to be accompanied by a sustained increased expression of TNF-α in the reproductive tract and the extent of TNF-α expression seems to be directly dependent on the severity of diabetes [18]. Studies in a number of labs and our experiments in diabetic mice [23, 27] revealed that they demonstrate a decrease in the pregnancy rate (the proportion of mated females which turned out to be pregnant), but not in the number of implantations per litter or a significant increase in the resorption rate. The claim that TNF-α can act as a mediator of diabetes-induced early pregnancy loss [18] was supported by our study [26], which revealed that severely diabetic TNF-$\alpha^{+/+}$ mice exhibit a significantly lower pregnancy rate than severely diabetic TNF-$\alpha^{-/-}$ females. Importantly, differences in the pregnancy rate were observed in these females tested on day 8 of pregnancy. However, the pregnancy rate in these mice tested on day 4 of pregnancy (existence of blastocysts in the uterus) did not differ and was comparable with that demonstrated by nondiabetic females.

Since in embryo transfer experiments the implantation rate of TNF-α exposed blastocysts was found to be comparable with that of control ones, one can suggest that the decrease in the pregnancy rate in diabetic mice was mainly due to some defects arising in the uterus. The observation that diabetic mice exhibited an 'all-or-nothing' response, i.e. a decreased pregnancy rate but not a decrease in the number of implanted embryos in litters of pregnant diabetic females, clearly supports such a suggestion. In parallel, it implies that such a total implantation failure might be due to a dysfunction of mechanisms which are critical for the ability of the uterus to become receptive to the blastocysts, allowing implantation. Studies addressing the role of LIF in reproduction imply that LIF represents such amechanism.

Indeed, it has been revealed [5] that LIF knockout mice produce normal blastocysts but implantation of the embryos did not occur. Reciprocal transfer experiments have shown that LIF null blastocysts transferred to pseudopregnant wild-type females developed successfully to term, whereas wild-type blastocysts transferred to pseudopregnant LIF null females failed to implant. Furthermore, LIF null blastocysts were found to be appropriately located in the uterine lumen but no morphological signs of implantation such as apoptosis in the luminal epithelium and decidualization of the underlying stroma were observed in $LIF^{-/-}$ uteri.

Thus, these results strongly suggest that the implantation failure in LIF-deficient mice was not due to some defects specific to the embryos but to those arising in the uterus and these defects resulted in the total loss of its receptivity. Because studies in diabetic mice suggest that early pregnancy loss in these mice might also be due to the total loss of uterine receptivity and that TNF-α can, at least partially, be responsible for this effect, the question arises of whether TNF-α has the potential to alter LIF signaling pathways.

Signaling between TNF-α and LIF

In the past dozen years, significant progress has been made in understanding the molecular details of cytokine-mediated signal transduction, suggesting a variety of mechanisms whereby TNF-α can alter LIF signaling pathways. However, all of these mechanisms function in a cell type-dependent fashion and here we mainly discuss those that may presently be expected to act in the embryonic vicinity.

LIF and TNF-α, as well as many other cytokines, have the potential to regulate the proliferation, differentiation and apoptosis of cells, which is realized through their interaction with specific receptors on the surface of target cells, which are coupled to intracellular signal transduction pathways.

LIF signaling is realized through the binding of LIF to the LIF receptor/gp130 receptor complex, resulting mainly in activation of the JAK family kinases, which, in turn, activate STAT (signal transducer and activator of transcription) transcription factors, in particular STAT3 [28, 29]. This LIF signaling pathway is abrogated by the SOCS (suppressor of cytokine signaling) and PIAS (protein inhibitors of activated STAT) proteins [30]. Also, LIF is able to stimulate the mitogen-activated protein kinase (MAPK) pathway and such activation may result in suppression of STAT3-mediated effects [29].

The importance of the STAT3 signal transduction pathway for the acquisition of receptivity by the uterus was demonstrated in a study in mice having a gp130 receptor, which was deleted for STAT binding sites [31]. These mice exhibited failure of blastocyst implantation. Also, there is evidence implicating STAT3 in the regulation of trophoblast invasiveness [32]. These observations and a number of other studies addressing the functional role of LIF signaling in the uterus [references in 33] led to the conclusion that, for implantation to be successful, not only the ligand, LIF, must be expressed in the uterus at the right time and right level, but also its receptors and the signaling pathways must be activated [33].

The possibility that LIF signaling may be affected due to alterations in TNF-α expression seems first to stem from data demonstrating that LIF gene expression in many types of cells can be induced by the TNF-α [34–36]. As to the uterus, it has been shown that TNF-α is able to induce LIF expression in human endometrial epithelial and stromal cells in a concentration- and time-dependent manner [37]. The expression of LIF in this organ is tightly regulated. In the murine uterus, LIF is expressed at the basal level in the glandular cells by the end of day 1 of pregnancy, sharply increases on day 4 of pregnancy and again declines to the basal level on day 5 of pregnancy [33]. In other species, the temporal pattern of LIF expression is, generally, similar to that observed in mice [references in 33]. In summary, the above observations seem to suggest that a sustained increased TNF-α expression in the reproductive tract of females exposed to stress can alter the temporal pattern of LIF expression. Such a suggestion seems to be supported by data [37] suggesting that the NF-κB transcription factor can be involved in mediating signaling between TNF-α and LIF.

Indeed, TNF-α is able to activate various signaling cascades, one of which culminates in the activation of the NF-κB transcription factor [38]. The functional role of NF-κB residing in uterine and trophoblast cells remains unclear [39]. Experiments in mice with null mutations in genes encoding members of the NF-κB family proteins or those encoding key proteins that regulate its activity revealed no embryonic death, which can be attributed to an implantation failure [references in 39], suggesting that NF-κB is dispensable for implantation during an uncomplicated pregnancy. At the same time, there is convincing evidence suggesting aberrant NF-κB activation as a key event in the pathogenesis of a number of diseases such as asthma, rheumatoid arthritis, diabetes, and some types of cancer [40, 41]. In the light of these data, studies should be mentioned which suggest that diabetes may lead to activation of NF-κB in uterine cells [17]. Some authors consider this event as the first response to mount a transient NF-κB-dependent antiapoptotic reaction. Not questioning this suggestion, we only want to point out that, as a positive feedback loop exists between TNF-α and NF-κB [38], this burst of NF-κB activity may also alter signaling between TNF-α and LIF.

In this context, it is worth mentioning that NF-κB by itself seems to have a prominent potential to modulate the LIF signal transduction pathway [28]. Thus, it has been shown that STAT binding sites are often in close proximity to binding sites for NF-κB and some other transcription factors and that NF-κB can both inhibit and promote STAT3 DNA binding [references in 28]. Also, the promoter region of the IL-6 gene contains NF-κB binding sites and expression of this cytokine, which like LIF belongs to IL-6-type family of cytokines and also potently activates STAT3, is also controlled by NF-κB [references in 28]. Finally, members of the SOCS family proteins, which act as inhibitors of JAK-STAT signaling, are induced by cytokines such as IL-2, GM-SCF and some others [references in 28], the expression of which is controlled by NF-κB [42]. Remarkably, in vitro studies [43, 44] suggest that TNF-α has the potential to induce the production of feedback inhibitors of the JAK-STAT signaling pathway such as SOCS-3 and SOCS-1.

It seems data presented above support the hypothesis that an alteration of LIF expression may be involved in the pathogenesis of TNF-mediated stress-induced early embryonic death.

Conclusion

To date, relatively little is known about molecular mechanisms underlying stress-induced early embryonic death. Data presented in this review seem to suggest LIF as a good candidate for further studies addressing this topic. It appears that these studies may also contribute significantly to our understanding of mechanisms underlying the function of LIF during normal pregnancy. Indeed, gene ablation experiments revealed a number of molecules acting in LIF signaling pathways, which seem to be dispensable for normal embryonic development [28, 33]. It is conceivable that studies in stress-exposed models make it possible to reveal the functional role of these molecules.

Acknowledgment

Udo R. Markert is member of an European Network of Excellence, entitled 'EMBIC' (Embryo Implantation Control), supported by the European Union (contract no. 512040).

References

1 Wilson JG: Current status of teratology: General principles and mechanisms derived from animal studies; in Wilson JG, Fraser FC (eds): Handbook of Teratology: General Principles and Etiology. New York, Plenum Press, 1977, vol 1, pp 47–74.
2 Clark DA, Arck PC, Chaouat G: Why did your mother reject you? Immunogenetic determinants of the response to environmental selective pressure expressed at the uterine level. Am J Reprod Immunol 1999;41:5–22.
3 Toder V, Carp H, Fein A, Torchinsky A: The role of pro- and anti-apoptotic molecular interactions in embryonic maldevelopment. Am J Reprod Immunol 2002;48:235–244.
4 Chaouat G, Zourbas S, Ostojic S, Lappree-Delage G, Dubanchet S, Ledee N, Martal J: A brief review of recent data on some cytokine expressions at the materno-foetal interface which might challenge the classical Th1/Th2 dichotomy. J Reprod Immunol 2002;53:241–256.
5 Stewart CL, Kaspar P, Brunet LJ, Bhatt H, Gadi I, Kontgen F, Abbondanzo SJ: Blastocyst implantation depends on maternal expression of leukaemia inhibitory factor. Nature 1992;359:76–79.
6 Terranova PF, Hunter VJ, Roby KF, Hunt JS: Tumor necrosis factor-α in the female reproductive tract. Proc Soc Exp Biol Med 1995;209:325–342.
7 Pasparakis M, Alexopoulou L, Episkopou V, Kollias G: Immune and inflammatory responses in TNF alpha-deficient mice: A critical requirement for TNF alpha in the formation of primary B cell follicles, follicular dendritic cell networks and germinal centers, and in the maturation of the humoral immune response. J Exp Med 1996;184:1397–1411.
8 Marino MW, Dunn A, Grail D, Inglese M, Noguchi Y, Richards E, Jungbluth A, Wada H, Moore M, Williamson B, Basu S, Old LJ: Characterization of tumor necrosis factor-deficient mice. Proc Natl Acad Sci USA 1997;94:8093–8098.
9 Toder V, Fein A, Carp H, Torchinsky A: TNF-alpha in pregnancy loss and embryo maldevelopment: A mediator of detrimental stimuli or a protector of the fetoplacental unit? J Assist Reprod Genet 2003;20:73–81.
10 Chaouat G, Menu E, Wegmann TG: Role of lymphokines of the CSF family and of TNF, gamma interferon and IL-2 in placental growth and fetal survival studied in two murine models of spontaneous resorptions; in Chaouat G, Mowbray JF (eds): Cellular and Molecular Biology of the Maternal-Fetal Relationship. Paris, INSERM/John Libbey Eurotext, 1991, pp 91–104.
11 Tangri S, Raghupathy R: Expression of cytokines in placentas of mice undergoing immunologically mediated spontaneous fetal resorptions. Biol Reprod 1993;49:850–856.
12 Raghupathy R: Pregnancy: Success and failure within the Th1/Th2/Th3 paradigm. Semin Immunol 2001;13:219–227.
13 Pampfer S, Wuu YD, Vanderheyden I, De Hertogh R: Expression of tumor necrosis factor-alpha (TNF alpha) receptors and selective effect of TNF alpha on the inner cell mass in mouse blastocysts. Endocrinology 1994;134:206–212.
14 Pampfer S, Vanderheyden I, McCracken JE, Vesela J, De Hertogh R: Increased cell death in rat blastocysts exposed to maternal diabetes in utero and to high glucose or tumor necrosis factor-alpha in vitro. Development 1997;124:4827–4836.
15 Wuu YD, Pampfer S, Becquet P, Vanderheyden I, Lee KH, De Hertogh R: Tumor necrosis factor α decreases the viability of mouse bla stocysts in vitro and in vivo. Biol Reprod 1999;60:479–483.
16 Soto P, Natzke RP, Hansen PJ: Actions of tumor necrosis factor-alpha on oocyte maturation and embryonic development in cattle. Am J Reprod Immunol 2003;50:380–388.

17 Pampfer S, Cordi S, Cikos S, Picry B, Vanderheyden I, Hertogh RD: Activation of nuclear factor kappaB and induction of apoptosis by tumor necrosis factor-alpha in the mouse uterine epithelial WEG-1 cell line. Biol Reprod 2000;63:879–886.
18 Pampfer S: Dysregulation of the cytokine network in the uterus of the diabetic rat. Am J Reprod Immunol 2001;45:375–381.
19 Monzon-Bordonaba F, Vadillo-Ortega F, Feinberg RF: Modulation of trophoblast function by tumor necrosis factor-alpha: A role in pregnancy establishment and maintenance? Am J Obstet Gynecol 2002;187:1574–1580.
20 Gorivodsky M, Zemliak I, Orenstein H, Savion S, Fein A, Torchinsky A, Toder V: Tumor necrosis factor alpha mRNA and protein expression in the uteroplacental unit of mice with pregnancy loss. J Immunol 1998;160:4280–4288.
21 Gendron RL, Nestel FP, Lapp WS, Baines MG: Lipopolysaccharide-induced fetal resorption in mice is associated with the intrauterine production of tumor necrosis factor-alpha. J Reprod Fertil 1990;90:395–402.
22 Arck PC, Meroli FS, Manuel J, Chaouat G, Clark DA: Stress-triggered abortion: Inhibition of protective suppression and promotion of tumor necrosis factor-α (TNF-α) release as a mechanism triggering resorptions in mice. Am J Reprod Immunol 1995;33:74–80.
23 Torchinsky A, Toder V, Carp H, Orenstein H, Fein A: In vivo evidence for the existence of a threshold for hyperglycemia-induced major fetal malformations: Relevance to the etiology of diabetic teratogenesis. Early Pregnancy 1997;3:27–33.
24 Fein A, Kostina E, Savion S, Orenstein H, Shepshelovich J, Ornoy A, Torchinsky A, Toder V: Expression of tumor necrosis factor-α in the uteroplacental unit of diabetic mice: Effect of maternal immunopotentiation. Am J Reprod Immunol 2001;46:161–168.
25 Ito K, Karasawa M, Kawano T, Akasaka T, Koseki H, Akutsu Y, Kondo E, Sekiya S, Sekikawa K, Harada M, Yamashita M, Nakayama T, Taniguchi M: Involvement of decidual Valpha14 NKT cells in abortion. Proc Natl Acad Sci USA 2000;97:740–744.
26 Torchinsky A, Gongadze M, Orenstein H, Savion S, Fein A, Toder V: TNF-alpha acts to prevent occurrence of malformed fetuses in diabetic mice. Diabetologia 2004;47:132–139.
27 Machado AF, Zimmerman EF, Hovland DN, Weiss R, Collins MD: Diabetic embryopathy in C57BL/6J mice. Altered fetal sex ratio and impact of the splotch allele. Diabetes 2001;50: 1193–1199.
28 Heinrich PC, Behrmann I, Haan S, Hermanns HM, Muller-Newen G, Schaper F: Principles of interleukin (IL)-6-type cytokine signalling and its regulation. Biochem J 2003;374:1–20.
29 Ernst M, Jenkins BJ: Acquiring signalling specificity from the cytokine receptor gp130. Trends Genet 2004;20:23–32.
30 Horvath CM: STAT proteins and transcriptional responses to extracellular signals. Trends Biochem Sci 2000;25:496–502.
31 Ernst M, Inglese M, Waring P, Campbell IK, Bao S, Clay FJ, Alexander WS, Wicks IP, Tarlinton DM, Novak U, Heath JK, Dunn AR: Defective gp130-mediated signal transducer and activator of transcription (STAT) signaling results in degenerative joint disease, gastrointestinal ulceration, and failure of uterine implantation. J Exp Med 2001;194:189–203.
32 Corvinus FM, Fitzgerald JS, Friedrich K, Markert UR: Evidence for a correlation between trophoblast invasiveness and STAT3 activity. Am J Reprod Immunol 2003;50:316–321.
33 Cheng JG, Rodriguez CI, Stewart CL: Control of uterine receptivity and embryo implantation by steroid hormone regulation of LIF production and LIF receptor activity: Towards a molecular understanding of 'the window of implantation'. Rev Endocr Metab Disord 2002;3:119–126.
34 Hamilton JA, Waring PM, Filonzi EL: Induction of leukemia inhibitory factor in human synovial fibroblasts by IL-1 and tumor necrosis factor-alpha. J Immunol 1993;150:1496–1502.
35 Aloisi F, Rosa S, Testa U, Bonsi P, Russo G, Peschle C, Levi G: Regulation of leukemia inhibitory factor synthesis in cultured human astrocytes. J Immunol 1994;152:5022–5031.
36 Lorenzo JA, Jastrzebski SL, Kalinowski JF, Downie E, Korn JH: Tumor necrosis factor alpha stimulates production of leukemia inhibitory factor in human dermal fibroblast cultures. Clin Immunol Immunopathol 1994;70:260–265.

37 Laird SM, Tuckerman EM, Cork BA, Li TC: Expression of nuclear factor kappa B in human endometrium; role in the control of interleukin 6 and leukaemia inhibitory factor production. Mol Hum Reprod 2000;6:34–40.
38 Baud V, Karin M: Signal transduction by tumor necrosis factor and its relatives. Trends Cell Biol 2001;11:372–377.
39 Torchinsky A, Toder V: To die or not to die: The function of the transcription factor NF-kappaB in embryos exposed to stress. Am J Reprod Immunol 2004;51:138–143.
40 Karin M, Cao Y, Greten FR, Li ZW: NF-kappaB in cancer: From innocent bystander to major culprit. Nat Rev Cancer 2002;2:301–310.
41 Makarov SS: NF-kappaB as a therapeutic target in chronic inflammation: Recent advances. Mol Med Today 2000;6:441–448.
42 Li X, Stark GR: NFkappaB-dependent signaling pathways. Exp Hematol 2002;30:285–296.
43 Fasshauer M, Klein J, Lossner U, Paschke R: Isoproterenol is a positive regulator of the suppressor of cytokine signaling-3 gene expression in 3T3-L1 adipocytes. J Endocrinol 2002;175:727–733.
44 Fasshauer M, Kralisch S, Klier M, Lossner U, Bluher M, Klein J, Paschke R: Insulin resistance-inducing cytokines differentially regulate SOCS mRNA expression via growth factor- and Jak/Stat-signaling pathways in 3T3-L1 adipocytes. J Endocrinol 2004;181:129–138.

A. Torchinsky
Department of Cell and Developmental Biology, Sackler School of Medicine
Tel Aviv University, Ramat Aviv, Tel Aviv 69978 (Israel)
Tel. +972 3 6409626, Fax +972 3 6406149, E-Mail arkadyt@ post.tau.ac.il

Markert UR (ed): Immunology of Pregnancy.
Chem Immunol Allergy. Basel, Karger, 2005, vol 89, pp 72–83

HLA Class I/NK Cell Receptor Interaction in Early Human Decidua basalis: Possible Functional Consequences

Magali Rabot[a], Julie Tabiasco[a], Beata Polgar[a], Maryse Aguerre-Girr[a], Alain Berrebi[a,b], Armand Bensussan[c], Natasa Strbo[d], Daniel Rukavina[d], Philippe Le Bouteiller[a]

[a]INSERM U563, Hôpital Purpan and [b]Department of Obstetrics and Gynecology, Hôpital Paule de Viguier, Toulouse, and [c]Faculté de Médecine de Créteil, INSERM 659, Créteil, France; [d]Department of Physiology and Immunology, Medical Faculty, University of Rijeka, Rijeka, Croatia

Abstract

Human decidual NK (dNK) cells differ from their peripheral blood (PB)-NK counterparts. The major subset of PB-NK is CD56dim, CD16+, CD160+ (highly cytolytic), whereas the major subpopulation of dNK is CD56bright, CD16– and CD160– (high cytokine producer). Extravillous cytotrophoblast invading the decidua basalis in early pregnancy expresses the polymorphic HLA-C, and nonpolymorphic HLA-E and HLA-G molecules that can interact with specific HLA class I-dependent dNK receptors, including the immunoglobulin-like KIRs, the lectin-like CD94/NKG2 and the CD160 receptors. There is no clear evidence thus far that dNK cells kill trophoblast cells. Instead they are able to secrete cytokines which are likely to be beneficial for the placental development, maternal uterine spiral arteries remodeling, and the antiviral immune response.

Introduction

Natural killer (NK) cells are a class of lymphocytes involved in the innate immunity, providing an important first line of immune surveillance. They are characterized by the expression of CD56, an isoform of the NCAM adhesion molecule, and the absence of CD3 [1]. NK cells express a broad variety of activating receptors that, upon ligation with their specific ligands expressed on or secreted by target cells, triggered cytotoxic activity and/or cytokine and chemokine production [2]. To prevent unwanted reactivity, NK cells also express various inhibitory receptors, most of which are HLA class I-dependent [3]. Such inhibitory receptors control activation signals mediated by activating receptors [2, 4]. The consequences of NK cell activation are target cell lysis and/or the production of inflammatory cytokines, such as TNF-α and IFN-γ. NK cell effector functions limit viral infection and tumor burden. NK cells are found in peripheral blood (PB; they constitute ~10–15% of the lymphocytes) in secondary lymphoid organs from which they can migrate to infected or inflammatory sites in vivo [5]. NK cells were also found in the nonpregnant endometrium where their number varies according to the ovarian cycle [3]. NK cells are also massively recruited at the embryonic site of implantation, constituting the dominant cell type of maternal immune cells in the decidua basalis in early pregnancy [6]. Their numbers then decrease from mid-gestation onwards [3]. They are phenotypically and functionally different from their PB-NK counterparts. Such decidual NK cells (dNK) are in close contact with invading extravillous cytotrophoblast which migrates deeply into the myometrium and maternal spiral arteries, replacing the endothelial cells lining these vessels [7]. Such a massive presence of dNK cells at the maternal-fetal interface is intriguing and strongly suggests important functions.

Unique Subsets of dNK Cells

The intense expression of the CD56 NK cell markcr together with the absence of CD3 confirmed the NK nature of these decidual cells [3]. However, dNK cells are phenotypically and functionally different from their PB-NK counterparts. They differ from PB-NK cells in many ways. First, they differ quantitatively, as 15% of circulating lymphocytes are NK cells, whereas in decidua NK cells represent ~70% of the total immune cells. Second, it was found recently that around 3% of 10,000 genes studied by microarrays showed a significantly different expression in PB-NK and dNK cells [8]. Third, different subpopulations of NK cells defined by their CD56, CD16 and CD160 expression also differ between PB-NK and dNK cells (fig. 1). PB-NK cells contain two different subsets namely CD56dim and CD56bright constituting ~90 and ~10%, respectively. The major subset (CD56dim) which consists mainly of killer cells is also CD16+, CD160+ and perforin+ [9]. CD16 is a low affinity receptor for FcRIII, responsible for antibody-dependent cellular cytotoxicity [10]. The BY55/CD160 receptor is a MHC class I-dependent glycosylphosphatidylinositol-anchored (GPI) molecule [11, 12]. CD160+ cells have a high cytotoxic potential, do not

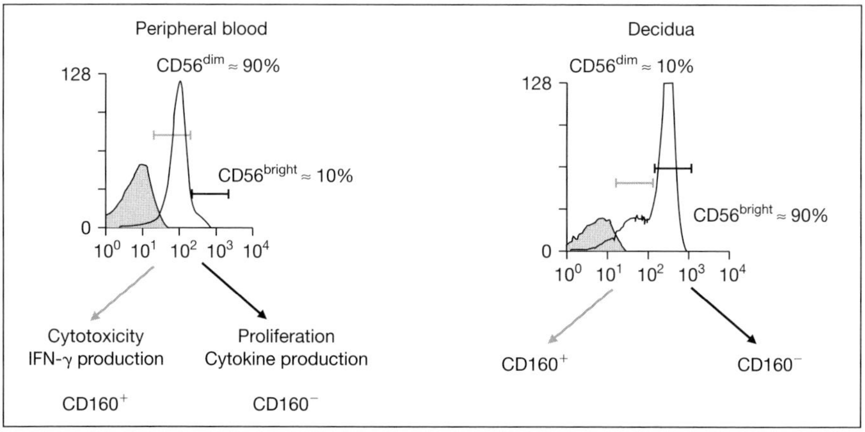

Fig. 1. Comparative flow cytometry analysis of CD56/CD160-expressing subsets between human PB (***a***) and dNK (***b***) cells.

proliferate in response to IL-2, and mediate lysis upon interaction with HLA-C [13]. Upon specific triggering of CD160, PB-NK cells also produce IFN-γ, TNF-α and IL-6 [14]. The minor PB-NK subset is CD56bright and is mainly a cytokine producer. This subpopulation expresses low levels or no CD16, and is CD160–. It is a proliferative and high cytokine producer NK population. In contrast to PB-NK, the major dNK cell subset is CD56bright, CD16– [3] and CD160– [Le Bouteiller et al., unpubl. data]. Only a minor dNK subpopulation is CD56dim and CD160+ (fig. 1). There are morphological differences between the PB-NK and dNK CD56bright cells. All the CD56bright PB-NK cells are small and agranular whereas most CD56bright dNK are large granular lymphocytes [15].

All these differences between PB-NK and dNK strongly suggest that they could exert distinct functions, the latter being possibly more dedicated to the placental development and pregnancy outcome.

Unique HLA Class I Expression of Fetal-Derived Invading Extravillous Cytotrophoblast

Extravillous cytotrophoblasts which invade the decidua are among the few somatic cell types which are devoid of classical HLA-A and HLA-B class I expression [16]. Among the polymorphic classical class I molecules, they only express HLA-C, as β_2-microglobulin-associated bound forms and free heavy chains, both maternal and paternal alleles being transcribed [17]. They also express the nonclassical HLA-E, HLA-F and HLA-G class I molecules

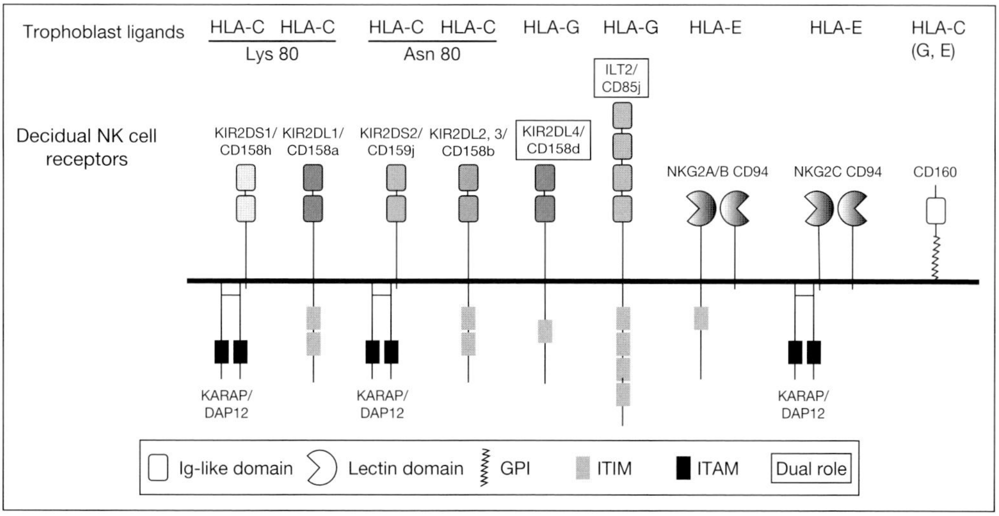

Fig. 2. Potential interactions between HLA class I molecules expressed by extravillous cytotrophoblast and HLA class I-dependent dNK cell receptors.

[16, 18, 19]. Several HLA-G isoforms have been described to date, including membrane-bound and soluble ones [20]. Membrane-bound HLA-G1 and soluble HLA-G isoforms, including soluble HLA-G1 and soluble HLA-G2, have been detected in extravillous trophoblast [21].

A Number of dNK Cell Receptors May Interact with Extravillous Trophoblast HLA Class I Molecules

Extravillous trophoblast cells intermingle with maternal immune cells at the implantation site in the decidua basalis, including the abundant NK cells, some antigen-presenting cells (macrophages, dendritic cells), CD4+ T cells and a few CD8+ T cells [22, 23]. A close association with endometrial stromal cells has also been described [24]. We will focus on the possible interactions between extravillous trophoblast HLA class I molecules and MHC class I-dependent receptors present on the surface of dNK cells. Such interactions are likely to occur since the extravillous cytotrophoblast attracts dNK cells by producing MIP-1α chemokines [25]. HLA class I-dependent cell receptors expressed on dNK cells comprise the following families of molecules (fig. 2).

(1) The killer immunoglobulin-like receptors (KIR). They possess various numbers of immunoglobulin domains and each member interacts with a particular HLA class I molecule expressed on extravillous cytotrophoblast cells, namely

HLA-C and/or HLA-G. KIR have both inhibitory and activating isoforms depending on the presence of inhibitory or activating motifs. Inhibitory KIR have one or two immunoreceptor tyrosine-based inhibitory (ITIM) motifs in their cytoplasmic domain which recruit and activate SHP-1 and/or SHP-2 phosphatases, thereby preventing downstream activating signaling cascades [26]. Activating KIR have immunoreceptor tyrosine-based activating (ITAM) motifs in associated molecules, such as KARAP/DAP12 [10]. HLA-C molecules are the ligands for inhibitory and activating KIR on dNK cells. Two major KIR epitopes have been described on the basis of a dimorphism at position 80 of the $\alpha 1$ domain [27, 28]. HLA-C^{asn80} is the ligand for KIR2DL2/3 inhibitory receptor and KIR2DS2 activating receptor, whereas HLA-C^{lys80} is the ligand for inhibitory KIR2DL1 and activating KIR2DS1. KIR2DL4/CD158d expression has been reported in both PB-NK and dNK. The putative ligand is HLA-G expressed by extravillous trophoblast. KIR2DL4/CD158d can act as activating receptor in resting PB-NK cells, inducing IFN-γ secretion but no cytotoxic potential, whereas in activated PB-NK cells the same receptor is capable of inducing cytotoxicity [29]. The activating signals sent by KIR2DL4 are sensitive to inhibition by other ITIM-containing receptors. However, a CD158d-null individual can successfully reproduce, suggesting that interaction between HLA-G and CD158d might not be so crucial for the pregnancy outcome [30].

(2) The Ig-like receptor ILT2/CD85j interacts with HLA-G, present on extravillous trophoblast [31, 32]. Although ILT2 contains ITIM motifs in its cytoplasmic tail, this receptor can exert dual inhibitory/activating functions [33]. ILT2 is expressed by 20–25% of dNK [18].

(3) The CD160 receptor is a cysteine-rich GPI-anchored receptor having an immunoglobulin external domain exhibiting a weak homology to the first immunoglobulin-type domain of KIR2DL4 [11]. HLA-C is a major ligand of CD160, triggering activating functions such as cytotoxicity and cytokine production [13, 14]. Although CD160 is expressed on a minor dNK subpopulation [34], the presence of HLA-C ligand on the extravillous trophoblast suggests that it can be activated.

(4) The C-type lectin family CD94/NKG2 heterodimers are composed of covalently associated CD94 and C-type lectin-like inhibitory NKG2A/NKG2B, or activatory NKG2C whose ligand is HLA-E. HLA-E molecules bind a peptide derived from the leader sequences of other HLA class I molecules [35], including those present on extravillous trophoblast (i.e., HLA-G, HLA-C). It should be noted that only the HLA-G leader sequence peptide complexed with HLA-E binds CD94/NKG2C with an affinity that is great enough to trigger an NK cell response [36]. So one can think that dNK cells could respond differently to extravillous trophoblast HLA-E compared to other maternal HLA-E expressing decidual cells which are HLA-G negative [6]. NKG2C and NKG2E

transcripts were found overexpressed in dNK cells [8]. The ligand, function and detection of NKG2E protein have not been reported yet. It was shown that most dNK were able to bind soluble HLA-E tetramer [37], suggesting that such interaction also occurs in vivo. Furthermore, it has been shown that the binding affinity of the inhibitory receptor CD94/NKG2A for HLA-E was higher than that of the activating CD94/NKG2C receptor [6].

Distinct Functions for dNK Cells in Pregnancy?

dNK cells express receptors for classical and nonclassical HLA class I which are expressed on the cell surface of or secreted by extravillous trophoblast. Exposure of dNK to fetal membrane-bound HLA-C, HLA-E, HLA-G and/or soluble HLA-G is likely to influence their cytokine secretion and/or their cytotoxic potential as well as their phenotype. It is still unclear whether such binding would block or activate cell lysis and/or lead to cytokine production that would control placental development, maintenance of pregnancy and contribute to preventing uterine viral spreading in case of infection. However, a number of observations indicate that such interactions have indeed functional consequences.

A recent important study reported that the combination of maternal KIR of AA genotype (lacking most or all activating KIR) with fetal HLA-C^{lys80} was associated with an increased risk of preeclampsia [38]. The authors hypothesized that this would be caused by an excess of dNK cell inhibition leading to poor trophoblast invasion and that an activating signal from maternal KIR is beneficial if HLA-C^{lys80} is presented by the fetus [38]. Further genetic studies performed by the same group showed that the addition of each activating KIR was associated with a 1.2-fold reduction in the prevalence of preeclampsia. This was the first observation that indicates a clear relationship between HLA-C molecules expressed by fetal extravillous trophoblast and maternal dNK cell KIR receptors. Another report extended these observations, indicating that 60% of the women tested who had recurrent spontaneous abortion were lacking the KIR2DL1 inhibitory receptor [39]. These authors further showed that a lack of KIR2DL1 resulted in a lack of epitope matching between maternal inhibitory KIR and fetal extravillous trophoblast HLA-Cw alleles in 33% of the cases. Such a lack of matching may predispose to miscarriage. The results presented in these two studies are in accordance with previous observations showing that more dNK cells than PB-NK cells did express KIR specific for HLA-C [38]. Overall, knowing that preeclampsia is characterized by defects in trophoblast invasion and maternal vascular remodeling, these results suggest that the interaction between maternal KIR and fetal HLA-C molecules may have important nonimmune functional consequences.

dNK Cells Are Very Unlikely to Play a Role in Cytotoxicity

So far, there is no clear evidence that dNK cells have a cytotoxic potential and are able to exert this function. Instead, a number of observations strongly support an absence of cytotoxic effects, contrasting with the major CD56dim PB-NK cell subset:

(1) dNK cells exhibit a noncytotoxic phenotype: they are CD56bright, CD16–, and CD160–. The CD56bright PB-NK cell subpopulation has a low cytotoxic potential. CD16 is expressed on the major CD56dim PB-NK subpopulation but is not present on dNK during early pregnancy [40]. This may be a factor explaining the low cytotoxicity of dNK cells. dNK cells also lack another marker of cytotoxicity, namely CD160 [13]. Despite the fact that granzyme B and perforin have been detected at similar RNA levels in dNK and CD56dim PB-NK, and that granzyme A is overexpressed in dNK versus PB-NK [8], dNK cells have a low potential cytotoxic effect on K562 target cells [3]. Thus, although a cytolytic potential does exist in dNK [41], it is likely to be controlled by unknown mechanisms.

(2) It is possible that extravillous trophoblast cells do not express enough triggering ligands of activating NK receptors such as NKG2D and natural cytotoxicity receptors. Indeed it has been shown that NKp30, 2B4 and NKG2D were not involved in the PB-NK cell-mediated killing of JEG-3 or JAR choriocarcinoma cell lines [42].

(3) Trophoblast cells are very resistant to cell lysis [43], unless dNK have been stimulated by IL-2 [44]. However, IL-2 is not present in the decidua. A recent study demonstrates that such trophoblast resistance to apoptosis was the result of the expression of the X-linked inhibitor of apoptosis (XIAP) which prevents activation of caspases 9 and 3 [45].

(4) In situ, no evidence of trophoblast cell lysis in early decidua has been provided yet.

(5) dNK cells are exposed to progesterone at very high concentrations [46]. It has been shown that a mediator of progesterone called progesterone-induced blocking factor blocked the dNK lytic activity [47].

dNK Cells Do Produce Cytokines

Transcripts for various cytokines have been detected in CD56bright dNK cells, including M-CSF, GM-CSF, TNF-α, IFN-γ, TGF-β and leukemia inhibitory factor whereas only TNF-α and TGF-β1 have been detected in resting PB-NK [48, 49]. Furthermore, dNK cells produce cytokines that are not normally produced by PB-NK cells, including leukemia inhibitory factor [50], and angiogenic growth factors angiopoietin-2 [51]. Such cytokine production by dNK cells may fulfill a number of functions which are subject of debates.

The role of these cytokines in the control of trophoblast invasion has been questionable since uterine NK cells are present in species with no trophoblast invasion into the uterus [3]. Furthermore, human trophoblast cells are very resistant to cell lysis (see above). Furthermore, perforin-deficient female mice were found to reproduce as efficiently as normal control females [52].

Such cytokines may also influence trophoblast growth since receptors for GM-CSF, CSF-1, IFN-γ and TNF-α have been found in human trophoblast cells [49].

Their potential role in the control of uterine vascular remodeling has also been evoked. It is based on the elegant experiments performed by the group of Croy [53] in murine models. NK cell-deficient or IFN-γ-KO-pregnant mice exhibit abnormalities in their decidual vasculature including abnormal thickening of the spiral arteries. Such vascular defaults are rescued after injection of allogeneic NK cells or after murine or human IFN-γ [54]. The mouse model provides important information about the role of dNK cell cytokine secretion in early pregnancy. Whether such a role also occurs during human pregnancy remains to be demonstrated. Some observations suggest that it could be the case. dNK cells are closely associated with maternal spiral arteries; they often form aggregates around them, possibly reflecting their trafficking from the circulation [55]. An increased production of IFN-γ and VEGF by dNK cells upon HLA-G interaction in vitro was recently reported [50]. Preeclampsia defaults of vascularization are associated with a lack of HLA-G expression [56].

NK cells play an important role in the early defense against viruses and also influence adaptive immunity to limit viremia. The cytokine production by dNK cells might be crucial to prevent possible viral spreading to the fetus in case of uterine infection by stimulating adaptive immunity. They might control cytomegalovirus spreading by secreting large amounts of IFN-γ [57]. It is striking that HLA-C, HLA-E and HLA-G trophoblast molecules are uniquely resistant to the effects of some human cytomegalovirus-derived US proteins [58–60] or HIV-1 proteins [61].

It should be noted that, in addition to the HLA class I-dependent receptors, some HLA class I-independent activating receptors, including natural cytotoxicity receptors, can also be expressed by dNK [62]. Such activating receptors are likely to be negatively controlled by the different HLA class I-dependent inhibitory receptors present on dNK.

Conclusion

Human dNK cells comprise distinct subpopulations in terms of phenotype and functions, which made them different from their PB-NK counterparts. It is likely that more functional dNK cell subsets will be defined in the future. Much remains to be done to precisely define their functions in terms of trophoblast growth, control of uterine vascularization and antiviral functions. As pointed out by Bulmer and Lash [3], it is also possible that dNK cell function varies in different areas of the decidua basalis, 'those cells which are in a perivascular position being exposed to a different microenvironment than cells distant from vessels'.

Acknowledgments

P. Le Bouteiller's and D. Rukavina's teams are funded by the EMBIC European Network of Excellence Grant No. 512040. Magali Rabot was funded by the Ministère de la Recherche, Julie Tabiasco by a postdoc fellowship from Organon and Beata Polgar by a postdoc grant from the Association pour la Recherche contre le Cancer.

Several authors of this manuscript are members of an European Network of Excellence, entitled 'EMBIC' (Embryo Implantation Control), supported by the European Union (contract no. 512040).

References

1 Moretta A, Bottino C, Mingari MC, Biassoni R, Moretta L: What is a natural killer cell? Nat Immunol 2002;3:6–8.
2 Moretta L, Moretta A: Unravelling natural killer cell function: Triggering and inhibitory human NK receptors. EMBO J 2004;23:255–259.
3 Bulmer JN, Lash GE: Human uterine natural killer cells: A reappraisal. Mol Immunol 2005; 42:511–521.
4 Chiesa S, Tomasello E, Vivier E, Vély F: Coordination of activating and inhibitory signals in natural killer cells. Mol Immunol 2005;42:477–484.
5 Ferlazzo G, Thomas D, Lin S, Goodman K, Morandi B, Muller WA, Moretta A, Münz C: The abundant NK cells in human secondary lymphoid tissues require activation to express killer cell-Ig-like receptors and become cytolytic. J Immunol 2004;172:1455–1462.
6 Moffett-King A: Natural killer cells and pregnancy. Nat Rev Immunol 2002;2:656–663.
7 Fisher SJ, Damsky CH: Human cytotrophoblast invasion. Semin Cell Biol 1993;4:183–188.
8 Koopman LA, Kopcow HD, Rybalov B, Boyson JE, Orange JS, Schatz F, Masch R, Lockwood CJ, Schachter AD, Park PJ, Strominger JL: Human decidual natural killer cells are a unique NK cell subset with immunomodulatory potential. J Exp Med 2003;198:1201–1212.
9 Maiza H, Leca G, Mansur IG, Schiavon V, Boumsell L, Bensussan A: A novel 80-kD cell surface structure identifies human circulating lymphocytes with natural killer activity. J Exp Med 1993; 178:1121–1126.
10 Lanier L: Natural killer cell receptor signaling. Curr Opin Immunol 2003;15:308–314.
11 Anumantha A, Bensussan A, Boumsell L, Christ A, Blumberg RS, Voss SD, Patel AT, Robertson MJ, Nadler LM, Freeman GJ: Cloning of BY55, a novel Ig superfamily member expressed on NK cells, CTL, and intestinal intraepithelial lymphocytes. J Immunol 1998;161:2780–2790.
12 Agrawal S, Marquet J, Freeman GJ, Tawab A, Le Bouteiller P, Roth P, Bolton W, Ogg G, Boumsell L, Bensussan A: Cutting edge: MHC class I triggering by a novel cell surface ligand costimulates proliferation of activated human T cells. J Immunol 1999;162:1223–1226.

13 Le Bouteiller P, Barakonyi A, Giustiniani J, Lenfant F, Marie-Cardine A, Aguerre-Girr M, Rabot M, Hilgert I, Mami-Chouaib F, Tabiasco J, Boumsell L, Bensussan A: Engagement of CD160 receptor by HLA-C is a triggering mechanism used by circulating natural killer (NK) cells to mediate cytotoxicity. Proc Natl Acad Sci USA 2002;99:16963–16968.

14 Barakonyi A, Rabot M, Marie-Cardine A, Aguerre-Girr M, Polgar B, Schiavon V, Bensussan A, Le Bouteiller P: Cutting edge: Engagement of CD160 by its HLA-C physiological ligand triggers a unique cytokine profile secretion in the cytotoxic peripheral blood NK cell subset. J Immunol 2004;173:5349–5354.

15 King A, Burrows T, Verma S, Hiby S, Loke YW: Human uterine lymphocytes. Hum Reprod Update 1998;4:480–485.

16 Le Bouteiller P, Sargent I: HLA class I molecules in the placenta: Which ones, where and what for? A workshop report. Placenta 2000;21(suppl A):S93–S96.

17 King A, Burrows T, Hiby S, Joseph S, Bowen JM, Verma S, Burrows TD, Loke YW: Surface expression of HLA-C antigen by human extravillous trophoblast. Placenta 2000;21:376–387.

18 King A, Hiby S, Gardner L, Joseph S, Bowen JM, Verma S, Burrows TD, Loke YW: Recognition of trophoblast HLA class I molecules by decidual NK cell receptor. Placenta 2000;21(suppl A):S81–S85.

19 Ishitani A, Sageshima N, Lee N, Dorofeeva N, Hatake K, Marquardt H, Geraghty DE: Protein expression and peptide binding suggest unique and interacting functional roles for HLA-E, F, and G in maternal-placental immune recognition. J Immunol 2003;171:1376–1384.

20 Bainbridge D, Ellis S, Le Bouteiller P, Sargent I: HLA-G remains a mystery. Trends Immunol 2001;22:548–552.

21 Morales PJ, Pace JL, Platt JS, Phillips TA, Morgan K, Fazleabas AT, Hunt JS: Placental cell expression of HLA-G2 isoforms is limited to the invasive trophoblast phenotype. J Immunol 2003; 171:6215–6224.

22 Le Bouteiller P, Blaschitz A: The functionality of HLA-G is emerging. Immunol Rev 1999; 167:233–244.

23 Kammerer U, von Wolff M, Markert UR: Immunology of human endometrium. Immunobiology 2004;209:569–574.

24 Dosiou C, Giudice L: Natural killer cells in pregnancy and recurrent pregnancy loss: Endocrine and immunological perspectives. Endocr Rev 2005;26:44–62.

25 Drake P, Gunn M, Charo I, Tsou CL, Zhou Y, Huang L, Fisher SJ: Human placental cytotrophoblasts attract monocytes and CD56bright natural killer cells via the actions of monocyte inflammatory protein 1α. J Exp Med 2001;193:1199–1212.

26 Vivier E, Daëron M: Immunoreceptor tyrosine-based inhibition motifs. Immunol Today 1997; 18:286–291.

27 Mandelboim O, Reyburn HT, Sheu EG, Vales-Gomez M, Reyburn HT, Rybalov B, Strominger JL: The binding site of NK receptors on HLA-C molecules. Immunity 1997;6:341–350.

28 Borrego F, Kabat J, Kim DK, Lieto L, Maasho K, Pena J, Solana R, Coligan JE: Structure and function of major histocompatibility complex (MHC) class I specific receptors expressed on human natural killer (NK) cells. Mol Immunol 2001;38:637–660.

29 Rajagopalan S, Fu J, Long EO: Cutting edge: Induction of IFN-gamma production but not cytotoxicity by the killer cell Ig-like receptor KIR2DL4 (CD158d) in resting NK cells. J Immunol 2001;167:1877–1881.

30 Gomez-Lozano N, De Pablo R, Puente S, Vilches C: Recognition of HLA-G by the NK cell receptor KIR2DL4 is not essential for human reproduction. Eur J Immunol 2003;33:639–644.

31 Gonen-Gross T, Achdout H, Gazit R, Hanna J, Mizrahi S, Markel G, Goldman-Wohl D, Yagel S, Horejsi V, Levy O, Baniyash M, Mandelboim O: Complexes of HLA-G protein on the cell surface are important for leukocyte Ig-like receptor-1 function. J Immunol 2003;171:1343–1351.

32 Shiroishi M, Tsumoto K, Amano K, Shirakihara Y, Colonna M, Braud VM, Allan DS, Makadzange A, Rowland-Jones S, Willcox B, Jones EY, Van Der Merwe PA, Kumagai I, Maenaka K: Human inhibitory receptors Ig-like transcript 2 (ILT2) and ILT4 compete with CD8 for MHC class I binding and bind preferentially to HLA-G. Proc Natl Acad Sci USA 2003;100:8856–8861.

33 Saverino D, Merlo A, Bruno S, Pistoia V, Grossi CE, Ciccone E: Dual effect of CD85/leukocyte Ig-like receptor-1/Ig-like transcript 2 and CD152 (CTLA-4) on cytokine production by antigen-stimulated human T cells. J Immunol 2002;168:207–215.

34 Pröll J, Bensussan A, Goffin F, Foidart JM, Berrebi A, Le Bouteiller P: Tubal versus uterine placentation: Similar HLA-G expressing extravillous cytotrophoblast invasion but different maternal leukocyte recruitment. Tissue Antigens 2000;56:479–491.

35 Braud VM, Allan DS, O'Callaghan CA, Soderstrom K, D'Andrea A, Ogg GS, Lazeti S, Young NT, Bell JI, Phillips JH, Lanier LL, McMichael AJ: HLA-E binds to natural killer cell receptors CD94/NKG2A, B and C. Nature 1998;391:795–799.

36 Vales-Gomez M, Reyburn HT, Erskine RA, Lopez-Botet M, Strominger JL: Kinetics and peptide dependency of the binding of the inhibitory NK receptor CD94/NKG2-A and the activating receptor CD94/NKG2-C to HLA-E. EMBO J 1999;18:4250–4260.

37 King A, Allan D, Bowen M, Powis S, Joseph S, Verma S, Hiby SE, McMichael AJ, Loke YW, Braud VM: HLA-E is expressed on trophoblast and interacts with CD94/NKG2 receptors on decidual NK cells. Eur J Immunol 2000;30:1623–1631.

38 Hiby SE, Walker JJ, O'Shaughnessy KM, Redman CW, Carrington M, Trowsdale J, Moffett A: Combinations of maternal KIR and fetal HLA-C genes influence the risk of preeclampsia and reproductive success. J Exp Med 2004;200:957–965.

39 Varla-Leftherioti M, Spyropoulou-Vlachou M, Keramitsoglou T, Papadimitropoulos M, Tsekoura C, Graphou O, Papadopoulou C, Gerondi M, Stavropoulos-Giokas C: Lack of the appropriate natural killer cell inhibitory receptors in women with spontaneous abortion. Hum Immunol 2005; 66:65–71.

40 King A, Loke YW, Chaouat G: NK cells and reproduction. Immunol Today 1997;18:64–66.

41 Rukavina D, Podack E: Abundant perforin expression at the maternal-fetal interface: Guarding the semiallogeneic transplant? Immunol Today 2000;21:160–163.

42 Sivori S, Parolini S, Marcenaro E, Millo R, Bottino C, Moretta A: Triggering receptors involved in natural killer cell-mediated cytotoxicity against choriocarcinoma cell lines. Hum Immunol 2000; 61:1055–1058.

43 Van den Elsen PJ, van der Stoep N, Vietor HE, Wilson L, van Zutphen M, Gobin SJ: Lack of CIITA expression is central to the absence of antigen presentation functions of trophoblast cells and is caused by methylation of the IFN-gamma inducible promoter (PIV) of CIITA. Hum Immunol 2000;61:850–862.

44 King A, Loke Y: Human trophoblast and JEG choriocarcinoma cells are sensitive to lysis by IL-2-stimulated decidual NK cells. Cell Immunol 1990;129:435–448.

45 Straszewski-Chavez SL, Abrahams VM, Funai EF, Mor G: X-linked inhibitor of apoptosis (XIAP) confers human trophoblast cell resistance to Fas-mediated apoptosis. Mol Hum Reprod 2004; 10:33–41.

46 Szekeres-Bartho J: Immunological relationship between the mother and the fetus. Int Rev Immunol 2002;21:471–495.

47 Laskarin G, Tokmadzic V, Strbo N, Bogovic T, Szekeres-Bartho J, Randic L, Podack ER, Rukavina D: Progesterone induced blocking factor (PIBF) mediates progesterone induced suppression of decidual lymphocyte cytotoxicity. Am J Reprod Immunol 2002;48:201–209.

48 Saito S, Nishikawa K, Morii T, Enomoto M, Narita N, Motoyoshi K, Ichijo M: Cytokine production by CD16–CD56bright natural killer cells in the human early pregnancy decidua. Int Immunol 1993;5:559–563.

49 Jokhi PP, King A, Sharkey AM, Smith SK, Loke YW: Screening for cytokine messenger ribonucleic acids in purified human decidual lymphocyte populations by the reverse-transcriptase polymerase chain reaction. J Immunol 1994;153:4427–4435.

50 Van Der Meer A, Lukassen HG, Van Lierop MJ, Wijnands F, Mosselman S, Braat DD, Joosten I: Membrane-bound HLA-G activates proliferation and interferon-γ production by uterine natural killer cells. Mol Hum Reprod 2004;10:189–195.

51 Li XF, Charnock-Jones DS, Zhang E, Hiby S, Malik S, Day K, Licence D, Bowen JM, Gardner L, King A, Loke YW, Smith SK: Angiogenic growth factor messenger ribonucleic acids in uterine natural killer cells. J Clin Endocrinol Metab 2001;86:1823–1834.

52 Stallmach T, Ehrenstein T, Isenmann S, Muller C, Hengartner H, Kagi D: The role of perforin-expression by granular metrial gland cells in pregnancy. Eur J Immunol 1995; 25: 3342–3348.
53 Croy BA, He H, Esadeg S, Wei Q, McCartney D, Zhang J, Borzychowski A, Ashkar AA, Black GP, Evans SS, Chantakru S, van den Heuvel M, Paffaro VA Jr, Yamada AT: Uterine natural killer cells: Insights into their cellular and molecular biology from mouse modelling. Reproduction 2003; 126:149–160.
54 Zhang JH, He H, Borzychowski AM, Takeda K, Akira S, Croy BA: Analysis of cytokine regulators inducing interferon production by mouse uterine natural killer cells. Biol Reprod 2003; 69:404–411.
55 Trundley A, Moffett A: Human uterine leukocytes and pregnancy. Tissue Antigens 2004;63:1–12.
56 Le Bouteiller P, Pizzato N, Barakonyi A, Solier C: HLA-G, pre-eclampsia, immunity and vascular events. J Reprod Immunol 2003;59:219–234.
57 Cooper M, Fehniger T, Caligiuri M: The biology of human natural killer-cell subsets. Trends Immunol 2001;22:633–640.
58 Barel M, Pizzato N, van Leeuwen D, Le Bouteiller P, Wiertz EJHJ, Lenfant F: Amino acid composition of $\alpha 1/\alpha 2$ domains and cytoplasmic tail of MHC class I molecules determines their susceptibility to human cytomegalovirus US11-mediated down-regulation. Eur J Immunol 2003; 33:1707–1716.
59 Barel MT, Ressing M, Pizzato N, van Leeuwen D, Le Bouteiller P, Lenfant F, Wiertz EJ: Human cytomegalovirus-encoded Unique Short 2 differentially affects surface expression of MHC class I locus products and targets membrane-bound, but not soluble HLA-G1 for degradation. J Immunol 2003;171:6757–6765.
60 Huddleston H, Schust D: Immune interactions at the maternal-fetal interface: A focus on antigen presentation. Am J Reprod Immunol 2004;51:283–289.
61 Derrien M, Pizzato N, Dolcini G, Menu E, Chaouat G, Lenfant F, Barré-Sinoussi F, Le Bouteiller P: Human immunodeficiency virus 1 downregulates cell surface expression of the non-classical MHC class I molecule HLA-G. J Gen Virol 2004;85:1945–1954.
62 Lewis BJ, Croker S, Newton DJ, Lennon GP, Johnson PM, Christmas SE: Natural killer cell receptor expression by human first trimester decidual granular leukocytes and T-lymphocytes. Am J Reprod Immunol 2002;48:103–109.

Philippe Le Bouteiller
INSERM U563
Bât. A, Hôpital Purpan BP3028
FR–31024 Toulouse Cedex 3 (France), Tel. +33 562 748 374
Fax +33 562 744 558, E-Mail phil.lb@toulouse.inserm.fr

Market UR (ed): Immunology of Pregnancy.
Chem Immunol Allergy. Basel, Karger, 2005, vol 89, pp 84–95

The Significance of the Women's Repertoire of Natural Killer Cell Receptors in the Maintenance of Pregnancy

M. Varla-Leftherioti

Immunobiology Department, RSA Clinic,
'Helena Venizelou' Maternity Hospital, Athens, Greece

Abstract

Large numbers of decidual natural killer (dNK) cells are in direct contact with the invading trophoblast and are considered to be important for pregnancy, since they can produce cytokines and other mediators involved in the control of trophoblast invasion, trophoblast differentiation, decidual artery remodeling and placental augmentation. The dNK cells are also the main candidate cells to attack trophoblast in cases of alloimmune abortions, where the fetus is 'rejected' by the pregnant woman. The function of NK cells is regulated by a balance between activating and inhibitory signals provided by their heterocladic receptor repertoire upon recognition of specific ligands, most of which are HLA molecules (HLA-C, HLA-G, HLA-E) expressed on invading trophoblast. It is a challenge to investigate abortions in regard to the receptors that dNK cells bear and the MHC molecules that the trophoblast expresses. Our studies in couples with recurrent spontaneous abortion as well as in random cases of abortion revealed that aborting women usually have a limited repertoire of inhibitory receptors of the KIR family (inhKIR), and that many of them lack inhKIRs specific for the fetal HLA-Cw antigens. We suggest that some spontaneous abortions are caused because of a limited maternal inhKIR repertoire and a lack of maternal inhKIR-fetal HLA-C epitope matching. Among the different interactions of NK receptors with their specific counterparts on trophoblast, the inhKIR-HLA-C interactions appear to be those mainly involved in the function of an NK cell-mediated allorecognition system in pregnancy.

Introduction

Natural killer (NK)-like cells (large granulated lymphocytes with the phenotype CD3–CD16–CD56+bright) are the dominant decidual cell population from the first stages of pregnancy [1]. Due to their increased presence and direct contact with invading trophoblast, they are considered to play an important role in the establishment and the outcome of pregnancy [2]. There is evidence that, after blastocyst implantation and decidualization, dNK cells are activated, they produce IFN-γ, perforin and other molecules, including angiogenetic factors, so that they may control trophoblast invasion through their cytotoxic activity, and also initiate vessel instability and remodelling of decidual arteries to increase the blood supply to the fetoplacental unit [3, 4]. On the other hand, they are involved in cytokine-mediated immunoregulation of the maternal immune response producing Th2- and Th3-type cytokines, which result in placental augmentation and local immunosuppression and immunomodulation [5, 6].

After IL-2 stimulation dNK-like cells can become like classical NK cells expressing CD16 (CD3–CD16+CD56+) [7], thus providing a population that can actually get involved in cytotoxicity and alloimmune reactions, where the fetus is recognized as 'foreign' and it is 'rejected' by the immune system of the pregnant woman (alloimmune abortion). Clinical studies have demonstrated that women who tend to abort have increased numbers of NK cells of the conventional CD3–CD56+CD16+ type in the uterus [8, 9], and increased blood NK subsets and NK cell activity have been associated with abortion of chromosomally normal embryos [10–12]. The triggering mechanism for NK cells to attack trophoblast has been an enigma, which can now be approached after all the new knowledge on the biology of NK cell that has appeared during the last decade and has illuminated many fields of immunology.

Biology of NK Cells and NK Cell Receptors

In the past, NK cells were considered to get involved in innate immune responses lysing infected and tumor cells without prior sensitization or MHC restriction. Today, it is known that these cells are not only direct cytotoxic killers, but that they also serve a critical role in cytokine production in order to control infections, cancer and fetal implantation [13]. It is also known that NK cell functions are tightly regulated by a balance between activating and inhibitory signals, transduced by distinct receptor types [14]. The NK cell receptors (NKR) belong to three main families: the KIR family (killer immunoglobulin-like receptors) [15], the C-type lectin family (CD94/NKGs) [16] and the immunoglobulin-like transcripts (ILTs or LIRs) [17]. All NKR families have both activating and inhibitory members. The activating members recognize specific, widely distributed ligands (including MHC class I molecules) on target cells, and trigger NK cell cytotoxicity after associating with molecules containing immunoreceptor tyrosine-based activation motifs (ITAMs). However, activation is controlled by the inhibitory receptors, which bear immunoreceptor tyrosine-based inhibition motifs (ITIMs) and deliver negative signals upon engagement to specific MHC class I molecules on target cells [18]. Human NK cells employ NKRs of all families for the recognition of different HLA class I molecules and the coexpression of multiple NKR combinations with specificity for different HLA alleles results in an effective regulation of immune responses. The NKR repertoire varies among individuals [19], and all mature NK cells express at least one dominant inhibitory receptor recognizing self-HLA class I products so that autoreactivity against normal host cells is prevented [20, 21].

The study of NKRs has provided important data indicating a possible involvement of these receptors in pregnancy. First, it was shown that an individual may express receptors for which he or she does not possess the relevant HLA class I ligand [22, 23], an indication that these receptors may potentially encounter nonself HLA alleles during alloimmune reactions, such as the host-versus-graft and the graft-versus-host reactions in allogeneic transplantation, and the maternal immune response against the semiallogeneic fetus in pregnancy. Then, it was demonstrated that dNK cells do express NKRs [24, 25], some of which appear to be selectively expressed on decidual cells [26]. More interestingly, the specific ligands for most NKRs are the only HLA molecules expressed on extravillous trophoblast (HLA-G, HLA-E, HLA-C) (table 1) [27–29].

Implication of NKR-HLA Interactions in Pregnancy

The importance to investigate the role of the interaction of dNK receptors with their HLA class I ligands on trophoblast was first emphasized in 1996, during a meeting on NK cells and reproduction, where it was suggested that Medwar's concept of 'the fetus as an allograft' needed to be redefined to encompass NK cells, and that the NKR-HLA interactions may provide a system that could explain several observations about the allorecognition at the fetomaternal interface [30]. This suggestion was a challenge for researchers to investigate the engagement of the different NKR members by specific HLA molecules expressed on trophoblast and the implication of these molecules for the function of dNK cells. In vitro studies have provided evidence for the involvement of NKR-HLA-class I interactions in the protection of trophoblast, although it was understood that the resistance of trophoblast to NK lysis also involves HLA class I-independent mechanisms [31, 32]. Most of the studies have focused on the interactions of the HLA-G antigen, which was thought to be a main factor for the protection of the fetus from dNK lysis, since its tissue distribution is restricted to the placenta. It was demonstrated that, although the protection of trophoblast from dNK cell lysis is not the main way for HLA-G to protect the embryo [33],

Table 1. NKRs and their MHC ligands

NKR	MHC ligand	
KIR		
KIR2DL1	(inh)	HLA-C allotypes Asn77, Lys80 (Cw2,4,5,6,15)[a]
KIR2DL2	(inh)	HLA-C allotypes Ser77, Asn80 (Cw1,3,7,8,12)[b]
KIR2DL3	(inh)	HLA-C allotypes Ser77, Asn80 (Cw1,3,7,8,12)[b]
KIR2DL4	(inh + act)	HLA-G
KIR2DS1	(act)	HLA-Cw4
NKG (CD94/NKG)		
CD94/NKG2A	(inh)	HLA-E[c]
CD94/NKG2B	(inh)	HLA-E[c]
CD94/NKG2C	(act)	HLA-E[c]
CD94/NKG2E	(?)	HLA-E[c]
ILT (Ig-like transcripts)		
ILT2/LIR1	(inh)	HLA-G (?), C
ILT4/LIR2	(inh)	HLA-G

inh = Inhibitory function; act = activating function; ? = unknown function.
[a] C2 group allotypes.
[b] C1 group allotypes.
[c] When specific HLA peptides (HLA-G1, HLA-C) stabilize HLA-E surface expression.

this molecule is a ligand for at least three inhibitory NKRs (table 1) [34–36], and that the expression of the HLA-G1 isoform as well other HLA-G truncated isoforms protects trophoblastic cells from lysis by activated NK cell clones [37, 38].

Implication of NKR-HLA Interactions in Abortion

In parallel to the in vitro studies, researchers started to investigate the function of the NKR-HLA system in the clinical setting of recurrent spontaneous abortion (RSA). As the HLA-C gene is known to be polymorphic, and the HLA-G and HLA-E genes have been shown to have a limited polymorphism, it was hypothesized that specific HLA alleles expressed on trophoblast could be inappropriate ligands for the engagement of the NKRs and the inhibition of NK-cell-mediated antitrophoblast cytotoxicity. However, the results derived from the comparison between fertile and aborting couples are conflicting. HLA-C and HLA-E polymorphisms were not associated with the outcome of pregnancy since no differences in allele frequency were found between aborting and fertile women [39–41]. As far as HLA-G polymorphisms are concerned, the results are contradictory. There are studies where no association was found [42, 43], and some others reporting an increased frequency of specific HLA-G alleles in aborting women, but there is no agreement between them on the alleles that are found to be increased [44–47].

Introducing a new approach to the investigation of the NKR allorecognition system in cases of RSAs, our team has focused on the NKR repertoire of aborting women and their partners. In a first study, we genotyped childless couples with RSA characterized by alloimmune abnormalities and fertile control couples for NKRs known to have as ligands HLA class I molecules, which are expressed on trophoblast: inhibitory 2DL1, 2DL2, 2DL3 and activating 2DS1 receptors of the KIR family (recogniton of supertypic epitopes shared between certain HLA-C alleles and HLA-Cw4, respectively), as well as inhibitory NKG2A and activating NKG2C receptors of the CD94/NKG family (recognition of HLA-E) (table 1). The comparison of the NKR repertoire between groups and/or partners revealed that any differences found concerned only the inhibitory KIR (inhKIR) receptors (2DL1, 2DL2, 2DL3), and that a significantly higher percentage of aborting women than women with successful pregnancies had a limited inhKIR repertoire and/or were lacking inhKIRs possessed by their husbands [48]. In an interpretation of our results, we hypothesized that a limited inhKIR repertoire may predispose to miscarriage and that some alloimmune abortions may occur because the MHC-C molecules on trophoblast are not recognized by dNK cells inhKIR receptors which would abort activating signals. To confirm this hypothesis, we investigated the specificity of women's inhKIR repertoire for the HLA-Cw antigens expressed on trophoblast in selected couples where the partners' HLA-C phenotypes consisted of antigens that are ligands for inhKIRs (Cw2,6,5,6 = ligands for 2DL2, 2DL3, Cw1,3,7,8 = ligands for 2DL1). Based on the HLA-C antigens of the partners, there was speculation about the four possible HLA-C phenotypes, one of which would be expressed on trophoblast, and it was estimated whether maternal inhKIRs had specificity for the HLA-Cw antigens of these phenotypes. The results revealed that 40% of the aborters did not have the appropriate inhKIRs to recognize ligands on all HLA-C phenotypes possibly expressed on the trophoblast [49]. To confirm this indirect finding, we analyzed epitope matching between maternal inhKIR and trophoblastic HLA-Cw allotypes in randomly selected women, who were undergoing vacuum uterine curettage for pregnancy failure in the 1st trimester or for elective termination of normal pregnancy. The samples taken via uterine curetting were used to extract DNA from isolated decidual and trophoblastic cells in order to genotype maternal inhKIRs (2DL1, 2DL2, 2DL3) and fetal HLA-Cw alleles, respectively. This new approach revealed that 60% of the women who experienced spontaneous abortion (vs. 6.6% in the women with elective abortion) did not have the full repertoire of 3 inhKIRs, all of them missing the 2DL1 receptor alone or in combination with other ihnKIRs. In

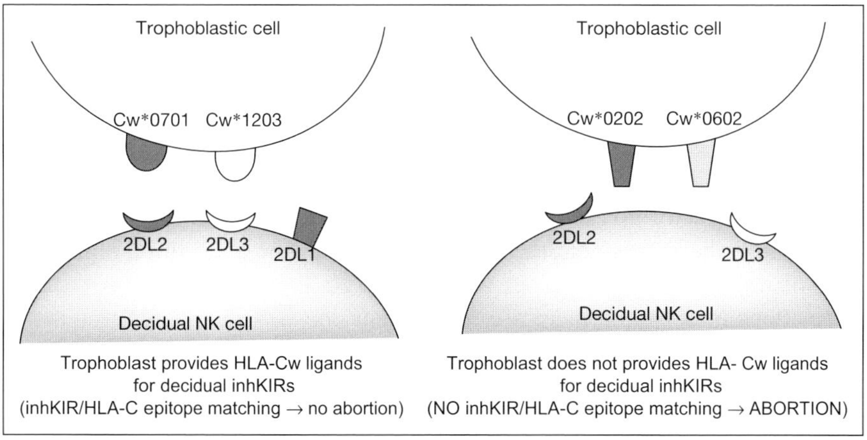

Fig. 1. Example of decidual inhKIR/trophoblastic HLA-Cw epitope matching (***a***) and no epitope matching (***b***) according to the inhKIRs that the mother possesses and the HLA-Cw alleles found on trophoblast.

addition, in 33.3% of the aborters (vs. 0% in the control group) no epitope matching existed between maternal ihnKIRs and trophoblastic HLA-Cw alleles, and more cases among them were found with a limited epitope matching (less than three inhKIRs with specificity for fetal HLA-Cw allele) [50]. Interestingly, it was observed that most of the aborters with a lack of matching had experienced repeated miscarriages and had no live birth.

Based on the above results, we suggest that the interaction of inhKIR receptors expressed on dNK cells with their trophoblastic HLA-C counterparts has a regulatory role in pregnancy, and it is involved in abortion (inhKIR/HLA-C allorecognition system) [51]. In cases where the women do not possess the appropriate inhKIRs to interact with trophoblastic HLA-Cw molecules, the triggering signals that the dNK cells may receive to attack the trophoblast (including activation signals provided through interactions of activating NKR-trophoblastic HLA-Cw pairs) are not inhibited, and the embryo is not protected. Thus, the detection of a lack of maternal inhKIR-trophoblastic HLA-Cw epitope matching in aborting women may indicate an immunogenetic etiology of their miscarriage, and similar to the above analysis could be useful in the investigation of women with unexplained RSA (fig. 1).

Importance of the inhKIR/HLA-C Interactions

Although the potential exists for dNK receptors to interact with trophoblastic HLA-I molecules, the way in which these receptors function in the outcome of pregnancy still remains unclear. Our suggestion for the implication of the inhKIR receptors and their HLA-C counterparts in abortion is an interesting hypothesis, which still needs to be confirmed by studies from other groups. Up to now, no similar analysis of maternal inhKIR-trophoblastic HLA-Cw epitope matching has been published, and in one recent study, where KIR polymorphism was investigated, no differences were found in the KIR repertoire (both inhibitory and activation KIRs) between RSA patients and controls [52].

Despite the absence of other studies confirming the implication of inhKIR-HLA-C or suggesting other specific maternal NKR-trophoblastic HLA class I interactions in abortion, there are several data in favor of the involvement of inhKIRs and their counterparts, HLA-C allotypes, in the recognition/rejection of the semiallogeneic fetus by the mother. For example, it has been demonstrated that in normal pregnancy the proportion of dNK expressing inhKIRs specific for HLA-C is increased, in comparison to that of peripheral NKs [23], and that this proportion decreases significantly in anembryonic pregnancies [53]. Furthermore, in a recent study, where the immunophenotypic characteristics of peripheral NK cells were investigated, a significant decrease in CD158a expression (2DL1) was demonstrated in RSA women as compared with that in controls [54]. On the other hand, there are no data suggesting an association of other KIRs or NKRs interacting with HLA-G and/or HLA-E with abortion. In our own study, where aborting couples were also genotyped for NKG2 receptors having a specificity for HLA-E, no difference was found in the NKG2 repertoire between aborters and controls [48]. Even for the interaction between the 2DL4 KIR receptor with HLA-G, which has attracted much interest because of the unique structural, functional and genetic features of 2DL4 and the restricted distribution of HLA-G to the placenta, it was demonstrated that it is not essential for pregnancy [55].

The control of the antitrophoblast activity of dNK cells during pregnancy is probably the result of the cumulative interaction of several NKRs on maternal dNK with different self and nonself class I molecules appearing on the HLA haplotypes expressed on trophoblast. However, inhKIR-HLA-C interactions are likely to have a predominant inhibitory effect, the absence of which may be a reason for abortion. An answer to the question of 'why inhKIR-HLA-C and not other NKR-HLA class I interactions?' must be given in regard to the polymorphism of both the KIR and HLA-C loci, which results in the expression of different HLA-C alleles and KIR genotypes in unrelated individuals. HLA-C locus is highly polymorphic, while HLA-G and HLA-E have a limited polymorphism [56]. The KIR genomic region also displays extensive polymorphism, both in the number of genes expressed in an individual and the alleles present for a gene, and inhKIR genes (2DL1, 2, 3) are among those KIR genes that can be absent or present on different haplotypes [19, 57, 58]. This is not the case for all KIR genes (KIR2DL4, which engage HLA-G, is present on most haplotypes) [57], CD94/NKG2 genes are generally conserved (only NKG2 genes exhibit some polymorphism) [57, 59], and, with the exception of ILT6, ILT genes do not exhibit a presence/absence variation [60]. Given the differences in both the inhKIR repertoire and the HLA-C allotypes among unrelated individuals, each pregnancy presents a different combination of maternal inhKIR receptors on dNK and self and nonself HLA-C allotypes on trophoblast. This combination does not always ensure the appropriate receptor-ligand interactions to inhibit dNK antitrophoblast activity, thus sometimes it favors abortion. The combined effect of the polymorphic maternal KIR and fetal HLA-C genes has also been demonstrated to influence the risk of preeclampsia and reproductive success [61, 62].

Apart from their possible involvement in abortion, inhKIR/HLA-C interactions have been suggested to contribute to the pathogenesis of other diseases, including disorders of human reproduction and autoimmune diseases. Overexpression of the KIR2DL1 inhibitory receptor on women's NK cells in peritoneal fluid and peripheral blood represents a risk factor in the pathogenesis of endometriosis [63, 64]. In rheumatoid arthritis, psoriatic arthritis and type I diabetes, the interaction of activating KIRs with HLA molecules in the absence of or during the downregulation of inhKIR/ligand pairs appears to facilitate autoimmune responses [65–67]. Finally, inhKIR/HLA-C interactions influence the success rate of hematopoietic stem cell transplantation. In leukemic patients who receive transplants mismatched for KIR ligands (absence in recipients of donor HLA-C allelic groups that engage inhKIRs), the donor-versus-recipient NK cell alloreactivity eliminates leukemia relapse and graft rejection and protects against graft-versus-host disease [68, 69]. This implication is similar to the suggested implication in abortion, given that the two situations involve allogeneic interactions, where KIRs specific for nonself HLA allotypes may meet their cognate ligands. In the case of hematopoietic stem cell transplantation, several groups have started clinical approaches to manipulate receptor/ligand interactions for clinical benefit, and search for the appropriate HLA class I mismatches to set NK cells in action [69]. In abortion, such a manipulation is not possible, but the inhKIR/HLA-C allorecognition model, if confirmed, could be used in the investigation of unexplained abortions.

References

1 King A, Burrows T, Loke YW: Human uterine natural killer cells. Nat Immunol 1996;5:41–52.

2 Clark DA, Arck PC, Jalali R, Merali FS, Manuel J, Chaouat G, Underwood JV, Mowbray JF: Psycho-neuro-cytokine/endocrine pathways in immunoregulation during pregnancy. Am J Reprod Immunol 1996;35:330–337.

3 Croy BA, Esadeg S, Chantakru S, van den Heuvel M, Paffaro VA, He H, Black GP, Ashkar AA, Kiso Y, Zhang J: Update on pathways regulating the activation of uterine natural killer cells, their interactions with decidual spiral arteries and homing of their precursors to the uterus. J Reprod Immunol 2003;59:175–191.
4 Trundley A, Moffett A: Human uterine leukocytes and pregnancy. Tissue Antigens 2004;63:1–12.
5 Chaouat G, Tranchot Diallo J, Volumenie JL, Menu E, Gras G, Delage G, Mognetti B: Immune suppression and Th1/Th2 balance in pregnancy revisited: A (very) personal tribute to Tom Wegmann. Am J Immunol 1997;37:427–434.
6 Clark DA, Croitoru K: TH1/TH2,3 imbalance due to cytokine-producing NK, gammadelta T and NK-gammadelta T cells in murine pregnancy decidua in success or failure of pregnancy. Am J Reprod Immunol 2001;45:257–265.
7 King A, Wheeler R, Carter NP, Francis DP, Loke YW: The response of human decidual leukocytes to IL-2. Cell Immunol 1992;141:409–421.
8 Vassiliadou N, Bulmer JN: Immunohistochemical evidence for increased numbers of 'classic' CD57+ natural killer cells in the endometrium of women suffering spontaneous early pregnancy loss. Hum Reprod 1996;11:1569–1574.
9 Kwak JY, Beer AE, Kim SH, Mantouvalos HP: Immunopathology of the implantation site utilizing monoclonal antibodies to natural killer cells in women with recurrent pregnancy losses. Am J Reprod Immunol 1999;41:91–98.
10 Coulam CB, Goodman C, Roussev RG, Thomason EJ, Beaman KD: Systemic CD56+ cells can predict pregnancy outcome. Am J Reprod Immunol 1995;33:40–46.
11 Aoki K, Kajiura S, Matsumoto Y, Ogasawar M, Okada S, Yagami Y, Gleicher N: Preconceptual natural killer cell activity as a predictor of miscarriage. Lancet 1995;345:1340–1342.
12 Yamada H, Kato EH, Kobashi G, Ebina Y, Shimada S, Morikawa M, Sakuvagi N, Fujimoto S: High NK cell activity in early pregnancy correlates with subsequent abortion with normal chromosomes in women with recurrent abortion. Am J Reprod Immunol 2001;46:132–136.
13 Miller JS: The biology of natural killer cells in cancer, infection, and pregnancy. Exp Hematol 2001;29:1157–1168.
14 Yokoyama WM: Recognition structures on natural killer cells. Curr Opin Immunol 1993;5:67–73.
15 Moretta A, Vitale M, Bottino C, Orengo AM, Morelli L, Augugliaro R, Barbaresi M, Ciccone E, Moretta L: P58 molecules as putative receptors for the major histocompatibility complex (MHC) class I molecules in human natural killer (NK) cells. Anti-p58 antibodies reconstitute lysis of MHC class I-protected cells in NK clones displaying different specificities. J Exp Med 1993; 178:597–604.
16 Lazetic S, Chang C, Houchins JP, Lanier LL, Phillips JH: Human NK cell receptors involved in MHC class I recognition are disulfide-linked heterodimers of CD94 and NKG2 subunits. J Immunol 1996;157:4741–4745.
17 Samaridis J, Colonna M: Cloning of novel immunoglobulin superfamily receptors expressed on human myeloid and lymphoid cells: Structural evidence for new stimulatory and inhibitory pathways. Eur J Immunol 1997;27:660–665.
18 Vivier E, Daeron M: Immunoreceptor tyrosine-based inhibition motifs. Immunol Today 1997;18:286–291.
19 Uhrberg M, Valiante NM, Shum BP, Shilling HG, Lienert-Weidenbach K, Corliss B, Tyan D, Lanier LL, Parham P: Human diversity in killer cell inhibitory receptor genes. Immunity 1997; 7:753–763.
20 Lanier LL, Phillips JH: Inhibitory MHC class I receptors on NK cells and T cells. Immunol Today 1996;17:86–91.
21 Long EO: Regulation of immune responses through inhibitory receptors. Annu Rev Immunol 1999;17:875–904.
22 Gumperz JE, Valiante NM, Parham P, Lanier LL, Tyan D: Heterogenous phenotypes of expression of the NKB1 natural killer cell class I receptor among individuals of different human histocompatibility antigens types appear genetically regulated, but not linked to major histocompatibility complex haplotype. J Exp Med 1996;183:1817–1827.
23 Verma S, King A, Loke YW: Expression of killer cell inhibitory receptors on human uterine natural killer cells. Eur J Immunol 1997;27:979–983.

24 Hiby SE, King A, Sharkey AM, Loke YW: Human uterine NK cells have a similar repertoire of killer inhibitory and activatory receptors to those found in blood, as demonstrated by RT-PCR and sequencing. Mol Immunol 1997;34:419–430.
25 King A, Hiby SE, Gardner L, Joseph S, Bowen JM, Verma S, Burrows TD, Loke YW: Recognition of trophoblast HLA class I molecules by decidual NK cell receptors – a review. Placenta 2000; 21(suppl A):S81–85.
26 Biassoni R, Bottino C, Millo R, Moretta L, Moretta A: Natural killer cell-mediated recognition of human trophoblast. Semin Cancer Biol 1999;9:13–18.
27 Kovats S, Main EK, Librach C, Stubblebine M, Fisher SJ, DeMars R: A class I antigen, HLA-G, expressed in human trophoblasts. Science 1990;248:220–223.
28 King A, Allan DS, Bowen M, Powis SJ, Joseph S, Verma S, Hiby SE, McMichel AJ, Loke YW, Braud VM: HLA-E is expressed on trophoblast and interacts with CD94/NKg2 receptors on decidual NK cells. Eur J Immunol 2000;30:1623–1631.
29 King A, Burrows TD, Hiby SE, Bowen JM, Joseph S, Verma S, Kim PB, Gardner L, Le Bouteiller P, Ziegler A, Uchanska-Ziegler B, Loke YW: Surface expression of HLA-C antigen by human extravillous trophoblast. Placenta 2000;21:376–387.
30 King A, Loke YW, Chaouat G: NK cells and reproduction. Immunol Today 1997;18:64–66.
31 Avril T, Jarousseau AC, Watier H, Boucraut J, Le Bouteiller P, Bardos P, Thibault G: Trophoblast cell line resistance to NK lysis mainly involves an HLA class I-independent mechanism. J Immunol 1999;162:5902–5909.
32 Zdravkovic M, Aboagye-Mathiesen G, Guimond MJ, Hager H, Ebbesen P, Lala PK: Susceptibility of MHC class I expressing extravillous trophoblast cell lines to killing by natural killer cells. Placenta 1999;20:431–440.
33 Bainbridge D, Ellis S, Le Bouteiller P, Sargent I: HLA-G remains a mystery. Trends Immunol 2001;22:548–552.
34 Madelboim O, Pazmany L, Davis DM, Vales-Gomez M, Reyburn HT, Rybalov B, Strominger JL: Multiple receptors for HLA-G on human natural killer cells. Proc Natl Acad Sci USA 1997; 94:14666–14670.
35 Moreau P, Paul P, Rouas-Freiss N, Kirszenbaum M, Dausset J, Carosella ED: Molecular and immunologic aspects of the nonclassical HLA class I antigen HLA-G: Evidence for an important role in the maternal tolerance of the fetal allograft. Am J Reprod Immunol 1998;40:136–144.
36 Le Bouteiller P, Blaschitz A: The functionality of HLA-G is emerging. Immunol Rev 1999; 167:233–244.
37 Pazmany L, Mandelboim O, Vales-Gomez M, Davis DM, Reyburn HT, Strominger JL: Protection from natural killer cell-mediated lysis by HLA-G expression on target cells. Science 1996; 274:792–795.
38 Menier C, Riteau B, Dausset J, Carosella ED, Rouas-Freiss N: HLA-G truncated isoforms can substitute for HLA-G1 in fetal survival. Hum Immunol 2000;61:1118–1125.
39 Christiansen OB, Mohapeloa HP, Steffensen R, Jersild C: HLA-C and -Bw typing of couples with unexplained recurrent miscarriages. J Reprod Immunol 1997;37:63–77.
40 Steffensen R, Christiansen OB, Bennet P, Jersild C: HLA-E polymorphism in patients with recurrent spontaneous abortion. Tissue Antigens 1998;52:562–572.
41 Kanai T, Fujii T, Keicho N, Tokunaga K, Yamashita T, Hyodo H, Miki A, Unno N, Kozuma S, Taketani Y: Polymorphism of human leukocyte antigen-E gene in the Japanese population with or without recurrent abortion. Am J Reprod Immunol 2001;45:168–173.
42 Karhukorpi J, Laitinen T, Tiilikainen AS: HLA-G polymorphism in Finnish couples with recurrent spontaneous miscarriage. Br J Obstet Gynaecol 1997;104:1212–1214.
43 Yamashita T, Fujii T, Tokunaga K, Tadokora K, Hamai Y, Miki A, Kozuma S, Jujii T, Taketani Y: Analysis of HLA-G polymorphism including intron 4 in Japanese couples with habitual abortion. Am J Reprod Immunol 1999;41:159–163.
44 Aldrich CL, Stephenson MD, Karrison T, Odem RR, Branch DW, Scott JR, Schreiber JR, Ober C: HLA-G genotypes and pregnancy outcome in couples with unexplained recurrent miscarriage. Mol Hum Reprod 2001;7:1116–1172.

45 Pfeiffer KA, Fimmers R, Engels G, van der Ven H, van der Ven K: The HLA-G genotype is potentially associated with idiopathic recurrent spontaneous abortion. Mol Hum Reprod 2001; 7:373–378.
46 Hviid TV, Hylenius S, Hoegh AM, Kruse C, Christiansen OB: HLA-G polymorphisms in couples with recurrent spontaneous abortions. Tissue Antigens 2002;60:122–132.
47 Abbas A, Tripathi P, Naik S, Agrawal S: Analysis of human leukocyte antigen (HLA)-G polymorphism in normal women and in women with recurrent spontaneous abortions. Eur J Immunogenet 2004;31:275–278.
48 Varla-Leftherioti M, Spyropoulou-Vlachou M, Niokou D, Keramitsoglou T, Darlamitsou A, Tsekoura C, Papadimitropoulos M, Lepage V, Balafoutas C, Stavropoulos-Giokas C: Natural killer (NK) cell receptors' repertoire in couples with recurrent spontaneous abortions. Am J Reprod Immunol 2003;49:183–191.
49 Varla-Leftherioti M, Spyropoulou-Vlachou M, Niokou D, Keramitsoglou T, Darlamitsou A, Tsekoura C, Papadimitropoulos M, Lepage V, Stavropoulos-Giokas C: Investigation of the role of the natural killer cell receptors' repertoire to the outcome of pregnancy; in Hansen J, Dupont B (eds): HLA 2004: Immmunobiology of the Human MHC. Proceedings of the 13th International Histocompatibility Workshop and Congress. Seattle, WA, IHWC Press, 2005.
50 Varla-Leftherioti M, Spyropoulou-Vlachou M, Keramitsoglou T, Papadimitropoulos M, Tsekoura C, Graphou O, Papadopoulou C, Gerondi M, Stavropoulos-Giokas C: Lack of the appropriate natural killer cell inhibitory receptors in women with spontaneous abortion. Hum Immunol, in press.
51 Varla-Leftherioti M: Role of a KIR/HLA-C allorecognition system in pregnancy. J Reprod Immunol 2004;62:19–27.
52 Witt CS, Goodridge J, Gerbase-Delima MG, Daher S, Christiansen FT: Maternal KIR repertoire is not associated with recurrent spontaneous abortion. Hum Reprod 2004;19:2653–2657.
53 Chao KH, Wu MY, Chen CD, Yang JH, Yang YS, Ho HN: The expression of killer cell inhibitory receptors on natural killer cells and activation status of CD4+ and CD8+ T cells in deciduas of normal and abnormal early pregnancies. Hum Immunol 1999;60:791–797.
54 Yamada H, Shimada S, Kato EH, Morikawa M, Iwabuchi K, Kishi R, Onoe K, Minakami H: Decrease in a specific killer cell immunoglobulin-like receptor on peripheral natural killer cells in women with recurrent spontaneous abortion of unexplained etiology. Am J Reprod Immunol 2004;51:241–247.
55 Gomez-Lozano N, de Pablo R, Puente S, Vilches C: Recognition of HLA-G by the NK cell receptor KIR2DL4 is not essential for human reproduction. Eur J Immunol 2003;33:639–644.
56 Schreuder GM, Hurley CK, Marsh SG, Lau M, Maiers M, Kollman C, Noreen HJ: The HLA dictionary 2001: A summary of HLA-A, -B, -C, -DRB1/3/4/5, -DQB1 alleles and their association with serologically defined HLA-A, -B, -C, -DR and -DQ antigens. Tissue Antigens 2001; 58:109–140.
57 Trowsdale J, Barten R, Haude A, Stewart CA, Beck S, Wilson MJ: The genomic context of natural killer receptor extended gene families. Immunol Rev 2001;181:20–38.
58 Middleton D, Curran M, Maxwell L: Natural killer cells and their receptors. Transpl Immunol 2002;10:147–164.
59 Shum BP, Flodin LR, Muir DG, Rajalingam R, Khakoo SI, Cleland S, Guethlein LA, Uhrberg M, Parham P: Conservation and variation in human and common chimpanzee CD94 and NKG2 genes. J Immunol 2002;168:240–252.
60 Young NT, Canavez F, Uhrberg M, Shum BP, Parham P: Conserved organization of the ILT/LIR gene family within the polymorphic human leukocyte receptor complex. Immunogenetics 2001; 53:270–278.
61 Hiby SE, Walker JJ, O'Shaughnessy KM, Redman CW, Carrington M, Trowsdale J, Moffett A: Combinations of maternal KIR and fetal HLA-C genes influence the risk of preeclampsia and reproductive success. J Exp Med 2004;200:957–965.
62 Parham P: NK cells and trophoblasts: Partners in pregnancy. J Exp Med 2004;200:951–955.
63 Wu MY, Yang JH, Chao KH, Hwang JL, Yang YS, Ho HN: Increase in the expression of killer cell inhibitory receptors on peritoneal natural killer cells in women with endometriosis. Fertil Steril 2000;74:1187–1191.

64 Maeda N, Izumiya C, Yamamoto Y, Oguri H, Kusume T, Fukaya T: Increased killer inhibitory receptor KIR2DL1 expression among natural killer cells in women with pelvic endometriosis. Fertil Steril 2002;77/2:297–302.
65 Yen JH, Moore BE, Nakajima T, Scholl D, Schaid DJ, Weyand CM, Goronzy JJ: Major histocompatibility complex class I-recognizing receptors are disease risk genes in rheumatoid arthritis. J Exp Med 2001;193:1159–1167.
66 Martin MP, Nelson G, Lee JH, Pellett F, Gao X, Wade J, Wilson MJ, Trowsdale J, Gladman D, Carrington M: Cutting edge: Susceptibility to psoriatic arthritis: Influence of activating killer Ig-like receptor genes in the absence of specific HLA-C alleles. J Immunol 2002;169:2818–2822.
67 van der Slik AR, Koeleman BP, Verduijn W, Bruining GJ, Roep BO, Giphart MJ: KIR in type 1 diabetes: Disparate distribution of activating and inhibitory natural killer cell receptors in patients versus HLA-matched subjects. Diabetes 2000;53:2639–2642.
68 Ruggeri L, Capanni M, Casucci M, Volpi I, Tosti A, Perruccio K, Urbani E, Negrin RS, Martelli MF, Velardi A: Role of natural killer cell alloreactivity in HLA-mismatched hematopoietic stem cell transplantation. Blood 1999;94:333–339.
69 Velardi A, Ruggeri L, Moretta A, Moretta L: NK cells: A lesson from mismatched hematopoietic transplantation. Trends Immunol 2002;23:438–444.

Dr. Marighoula Varla-Leftherioti, MD
Immunobiology Department, 'Helena Venizelou' Maternity Hospital
2 Helen's Venizelou sq, GR–11521 Athens (Greece)
Tel. +30 210 6453759, Fax +30 210 6402149, E-Mail gr1bmdr@hol.gr

Markert UR (ed): Immunology of Pregnancy.
Chem Immunol Allergy. Basel, Karger, 2005, vol 89, pp 96–104

Antigen-Presenting Cells in the Decidua

Ulrike Kämmerer

Department of Obstetrics and Gynecology,
University of Würzburg, Würzburg, Germany

Abstract

Maternal tolerance against fetal antigens is still one of the unsolved questions in pregnancy. Focusing on the various subsets of immune cells playing in concert with the human immune system, tolerance induction is nowadays often accredited to a specialized group of immune cells, the antigen-presenting cells (APC). There are surprisingly few reports about APC populations in the decidualized endometrium, the decidua where fetal cells get into contact with the maternal immune system. Nowadays it seems to be clear that at least three populations of APC, the macrophages, dendritic cells and immature, monocyte-derived APC, could be found in the decidua of a pregnant uterus. This chapter summarizes the characteristics of dendritic cells and macrophages as APC in general and focuses on the description and characterization of APC in the decidua of different species found in the literature.

Antigen-Presenting Cells in General

Antigen-presenting cells (APC) are critical players in the immune response. In order to fulfill their function as antigen presenters, APC serve two major functions. First, they capture the proteins from pathogens or cellular debris and process them in that they digest them into fragments called epitopes. Second, APC present these epitopes on either class I or class II major histocompatibility complex (MHC) proteins for T lymphocyte recognition. In addition to MHC presentation of peptides, APC express signals required for the proliferation and differentiation of T lymphocytes that specifically recognize the presented antigen. In general, APC are a heterogeneous group of immune cells, but traditional APC include dendritic cells (DC) and macrophages which are described in more detail below.

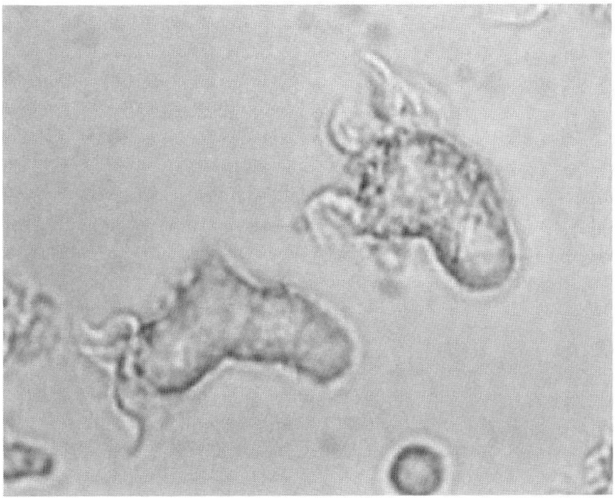

Fig. 1. Two DC isolated from human first trimester decidua exhibiting the typical DC phenotype with long dendrites extending from their surface and irregular body shape. Magnification ×1,000.

Dendritic Cells

DC are a heterogeneous population of bone-marrow-derived cells, yet they are the most potent of all APC. In vivo, DC exhibit a distinct shape, described as veiled or dendritic, with long motile cytoplasmic processes extending from their surface (fig. 1). DC express high levels of MHC class II on their surface and are able to migrate selectively through tissues [for review, see 1, 2]. DC pass through changing states of functional activity to optimally fulfill their mission; this is typical for APC (fig. 2). The first stage in their 'life cycle' is the so-called immature state; DC function as sentinels of the immune system. Immature DC are preferentially located at the surfaces of the body, throughout the epithelium of the skin, the respiratory tract, the gastrointestinal tract and the urogynecological tract, where they attach themselves via the long cytoplasmic processes. Upon invading pathogens and/or local tissue disturbance, resident immature DC are activated and together with additional APC are attracted by chemokines. The APC accumulate in the inflamed tissue and pick up antigens from pathogens or from dead cell debris through pinocytosis and phagocytosis [3]. Immature DC express several DC-characteristic adsorptive receptors mainly belonging to the lectin family. One of these monolectins is DC-SIGN (DC-specific ICAM-grabbing nonintergin, classified as CD209) which is a DC-specific adhesion receptor with a high affinity for the adhesion molecules ICAM-2 and ICAM-3. DC-SIGN can be found predominantly on immature DC and is capable of binding various antigens, for example the HIV protein gp120 [4]. Exogenous antigens are captured and internalized into the

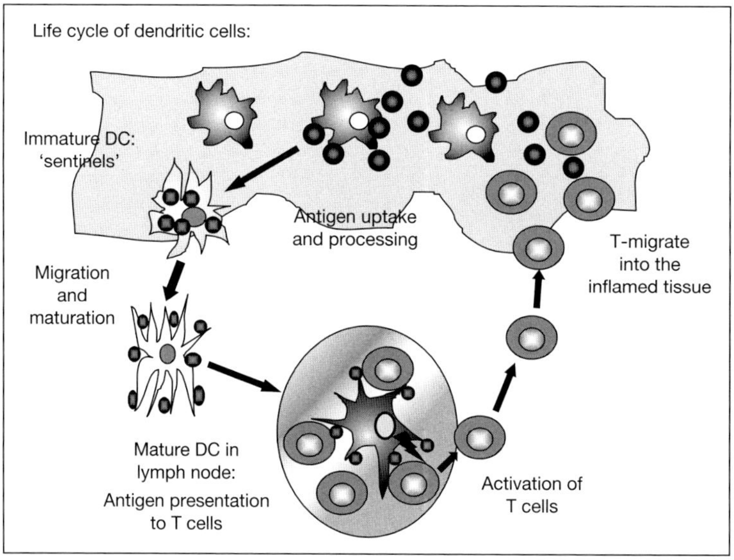

Fig. 2. Scheme of the life cycle of a DC. Immature DC placed as sentinels in a tissue get into contact with invading foreign antigen (e.g. infection; top). After uptake of antigens, DC migrate into the lymph vessels and undergo maturation (upper left). While migrating into the next lymph node, DC process the antigen into peptides which could then be presented on the DC's surface in a MHC-dependent manner (lower left). In the lymph node, the now fully mature DC loaded with the antigen in question select those T cells, whose receptor fit to the antigen presented. Via costimulatory molecules, these T cells were activated and start proliferation (bottom). The activated T cells will then migrate into the site of antigen invasion and attack the pathogens/foreign cells (right side).

endosomal compartments for processing of the antigen into peptides. DC become activated by proinflammatory cytokines like IL-1 or TNF-α and migrate from the site of inflammation via the lymph vessels into the regional lymph nodes. By the time they enter the lymph nodes, they have matured and are now able to present antigens to the ever-changing populations of naive T lymphocytes located in the cortex of lymph nodes. Mature DC have upregulated costimulatory surface molecules CD40, CD80, CD86 and CD83 and produce T cell-activating cytokines like IL-12. Therefore, they are potent immunostimulatory APC [5]. The last part of a DC's life cycle is terminating their antigenpresenting and T cell-stimulating activities by undergoing apoptotic cell death.

DC have long been studied to understand their capacity to activate T cell responses in vivo and in vitro [5]. However, in addition to their significant stimulatory capacity, DC have an important regulatory role in the immune system, including the induction of peripheral tolerance and regulation of the types of T cell responses. Concerning the function of DC as tolerance-inducing mediators, there is evidence that DC can be converted to Th2-skewing cells when treated with anti-inflammatory cytokines such as IL-10 [6] or glucocorticoids like dexamethasone [7]. There is further evidence that DC seeded on mucosal surfaces are responsible for the tolerogenic phenotype [8]. This may reflect a special DC subpopulation prone to act as 'tolerance inducing'. Thus, a similar subpopulation could be responsible for maternal tolerance against fetal antigens in the uterine mucosa, the decidua.

Macrophages

Macrophages are involved in almost all aspects of immunological and inflammatory responses. They seem to play an essential role in linking innate and acquired immunity Their main function is to phagocytose and destroy microorganisms and to kill virally infected and malignant cells. As APC, they present antigens to T lymphocytes. In addition, they play important roles in angiogenesis and tissue remodeling. Tissue macrophages are of a heterogeneous phenotype, because they adapt to the local microenvironment to perform a tissue-specific function [for review, see 9, 10].

There are relatively few markers that 'distinguish' between macrophages and DC, and the relationship between macrophages and DC has been a matter of as much debate as the original definition of the APC. Macrophages are derived from circulating monocytes which are attracted to migrate into tissues by chemokines/cytokines like the monocyte chemoattractant protein-1 (MCP-1). Under the influence of colony-stimulating factor-1 (CSF-1), the attracted monocytes proliferate in situ and differentiate into mature, nondividing tissue macrophages. Upon contact with antigens/microorganisms and under the influence of inflammatory cytokines the macrophages could be activated. This activation results in an increase in the production of toxic oxygen radicals, nitric oxide, and hydrolytic lysosomal enzymes. Furthermore, activated macrophages secrete cytokines such as TNF-α and IL-1, which promote inflammation to recruit phagocytic leukocytes, as well as IL-12, which enables naive T4 lymphocytes to differentiate into Th1 cells. The phenotype of activated macrophages changes in that a higher expression of B7 costimulator molecules and MHC-1 molecule expression increase T lymphocyte activation.

APC in Decidua

The precise mechanism by which the maternal immune system deals with fetally derived antigens during pregnancy is still not completely resolved. The requirement for APC to present antigens to lymphocytes make these cells an integral part for the induction of immunological responses. Therefore, it could be assumed that APC at the fetomaternal interface would be ideally located for presenting fetal antigens in a tolerance-inducing way. Endometrial tissue and the decidualized endometrium (decidua) in humans, nonhuman primates and rodents contain numerous leukocytes with the morphology and the phenotype of APC.

Early histochemical studies have shown a possible role for macrophages in the implantation on the rat uterus [11]. In contrast to the human uterus, where a remarkable population of early pregnancy human decidual cells was found to be HLA-DR+ by immunohistochemistry [12], macrophages were depleted from rat decidua shortly after implantation and therefore seem to only be important in implantation [11]. In 1984, Hunt et al. [13] demonstrated that macrophages from pregnant mouse uterus are immunosuppressive. Thus, they provided the first hints that APC may create a local environment prohibitive to maternal lymphocyte stimulation against the embryo. The first description of human decidual APC was published in the same year, when Bulmer and Sunderland [12] quantified HLA-DR+ cells in human decidua by immunohistochemistry and concluded that the HLA-DR+ cells in human decidua mainly belong to the macrophages. One year later, Elcock and Searle [14] described functional studies on isolated mouse decidua cells, which revealed at least two morphologically distinct populations of APC from day 8 till day15 of pregnancy. One of those APC populations was subsequently identified by Hunt et al. [15], who could identify a remarkably large population of mouse decidual cells as macrophages by immunohistochemistry with a rabbit-anti-mouse antibody raised against tissue macrophages. This immunohistochemical finding on mouse decidual macrophages was confirmed by Matthews et al. in 1985 [16], who used a rat monoclonal macrophage-specific antibody (F4–80) to demonstrate that a significant proportion of Fc receptor-bearing cells in the decidua were macrophages. One year later Oksenberg et al. [17] demonstrated 'dendritic-like Ia-positive cells' in human decidua that could be stained with the antibody 63D3 (macrophages) and were able to induce T cell proliferation. In the next publication on 'APC in decidua', Kamat and Isaacson [18] demonstrated using immunohistochemistry that macrophages (identified by UCHM1 and HLA-DR+) were diffusely distributed in the stroma of human endometrium. In 1988, Bulmer et al. [19] demonstrated that macrophages increase premenstrually and make up 35% of the decidual leukocytes around implantation. In the same year, Lessin et al. [20] performed a systematic study of HLA expression by human decidual cells throughout gestation. Like Oksenberg et al., they found a major (21–32%) proportion of maternal decidual cells with strong positivity for HLA class I and class II molecules. The class II+ cells were identified as macrophages by 63D3 staining. Also in 1988, Dorman and Searle [21] reported the alloantigen-presenting capacity of human decidual cells. Using the F4–80 antibody like Matthews in 1991, De et al. [22] demonstrated that, at the time of implantation, macrophages in the mouse uterus increase in number and are localized subepithelially to endometrial glands. Improvement in functional studies was seen in 1992, when Searle and Wren [23] managed to isolate decidual APC from whole-decidua cell suspensions via a plastic adherence step. In 1994, Mizuno et al. [24] described that isolated decidual macrophages are able to present soluble antigens in an MHC-restricted manner but also possess some suppressive activity for the maternal immune response. Contrary to these findings, Olivares et al. [25] described decidual stromal cells that by flow cytometry did not express the classical macrophage marker CD14, but did express HLA-DR as well as the activation markers CD80 and CD86. Since these cells were potent stimulators of allogeneic T cells, the authors were in favor of professional APC seeding the human decidua. The concrete nature of those decidual APC was not further characterized until 2000, when it was demonstrated that human endometrium and early pregnancy decidua harbors classical mature CD83+ DC, similar to those described for other mucousal surfaces [26]. Evidence for immature precursors of decidual DC was provided by Soilleux et al. [27], who detected DC-SIGN on HLA-DR+ decidual cells and described them as specialized decidual macrophages by their costaining for CD14 and the 'classical' macrophage marker CD68. In 2003, those DC-SIGN-positive decidual cells were then identified as precursors of immunostimulatory decidual DC by proving in vitro that isolated decidual DC-SIGN-positive cells can mature into classical CD83-expressing DC with high T cell-stimulatory capacity [28]. Also in 2003, Gardener and Moffet [29] identified a small (1.7% of decidual CD45-positive leukocytes) population of decidual DC expressing CD11c, a marker for myeloid DC, but none of the other classical leukocyte lineage markers. Confirmation of such a HLA-DRbright but lin– population of DC was given by Miyazaki et al. [30] who could clearly demonstrate by FACS analysis that human early pregnancy decidua contains lin– HLA-DRbright DC. Characterizing uterine DC populations in the mouse, Blois et al. [31] found the vast majority of uterine DCs to be of the myeloid lineage. Evidence for APC in the rhesus monkey was recently given in a report by Slukvin et al. [32], who found numerous CD64+/CD68+ macrophages in early pregnancy decidua in close association with invasive cytotrophoblasts. New data from the mouse uterus concerning macrophages were described by Lagadari et al. [33] who analyzed number and distribution of macrophages in placental tissue and found a significantly higher number of macrophages in multiparous than in primiparous mice. In a very recent publication, Askelund et al. [34] found a significantly higher number of mature DC in human decidual tissue from abortions than in normal pregnancies and speculated that mature DC may play a role in the pathophysiology of some cases of recurrent abortion.

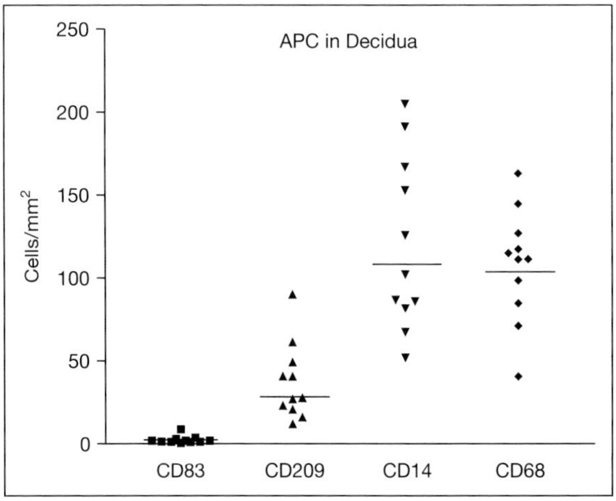

Fig. 3. Quantification of different APC populations in human decidua. From left to right there are mature DC as identified by CD83 staining, immature DC positive for DC-SIGN (CD209), CD14+ monocytes and classical macrophages stained with CD68.

In summary, different groups of APC populations are harbored in the decidua of pregnancy in the species investigated: classical macrophages, classical mature DC, immature/intermediate cells prone to mature into potent immunostimulatory DC (and perhaps macrophages?) as well as immature DC and myeloid DC (fig. 3).

The Functional Role of Decidual APC

The function of APC in the decidua is still far from being understood. It is very likely that specialized APC present fetal antigens (derived from the invasive trophoblasts) to the maternal immune system, but how this function of antigen presentation relates to inducing a state of tolerance to fetal antigens is unclear. It seems possible that the intradecidual microenvironment and cellular interactions decide whether APC will acquire characteristics and functions of classical antigen-presenting mature DC with T-activating features, or – more likely – arrest the APC in an immature or 'semimature' state which is thought to mediate tolerance induction [35]. In this respect, it is noteworthy that many of the factors described so far to promote tolerogenic DC are present in abundance in the decidua. Hopefully, further research on decidual APC will shed light on how these cells help to create the delicate balance between tolerance to fetal antigens and immunity to threatening agents.

References

1 Steinman RM: The dendritic cell system and its role in immunogenicity. Annu Rev Immunol 1991;9:271–296.
2 Hart DNJ: Dendritic cells: Unique leukocyte populations which control the primary immune response. Blood 1997;90:3245–3287.
3 Sallusto F, Lanzavecchia A: Mobilizing dendritic cells for tolerance, priming, and chronic inflammation. J Exp Med 1999;189:611–614.
4 Geijtenbeek TB, Torensma R, van Vliet SJ, et al: Identification of DC-SIGN, a novel dendritic cell-specific ICAM-3 receptor that supports primary immune responses. Cell 2000;100:575–585.
5 Inaba K, Metlay JP, Crowley MT, et al: Dendritic cells pulsed with protein antigens in vitro can prime antigen-specific, MHC-restricted T cells in situ. J Exp Med 1990;172:631–640.
6 Steinbrink K, Wolfl M, Knop J, et al: Induction of tolerance by IL-10-treated dendritic cells. J Immunol 1997;159:4772–4780.
7 Piemonti L, Monti P, Allavena P, et al: Glucocorticoids affect human dendritic cell differentiation and maturation. J Immunol 1999;162:6473–6481.
8 Weiner HL: The mucosal milieu creates tolerogenic dendritic cells and T(R)1 and T(H)3 regulatory cells. Nat Immunol 2001;2:671–672.
9 Van Furth R: Origin and turnover of monocytes and macrophages. Curr Top Pathol 1998;79: 125–150.
10 Burke B, Lewie CE: The Macrophage, ed 2. London, Oxford University Press, 2002.
11 Tachi C, Tachi S, Knyszynski A, Lindner HR: Possible involvement of macrophages in embryo-maternal relationships during ovum implantation in the rat. J Exp Zool 1981;217:81–92.
12 Bulmer JN, Sunderland CA: Immunohistological characterization of lymphoid cell populations in the early human placental bed. Immunology 1984;52:349–357.
13 Hunt JS, Manning LS, Wood GW: Macrophages in murine uterus are immunosuppressive. Cell Immunol 1984;85:499–510.
14 Elcock JM, Searle RF: Antigen-presenting capacity of mouse decidual tissue and placenta. Am J Reprod Immunol Microbiol 1985;7:99–103.
15 Hunt JS, Manning LS, Mitchell D, Selanders JR, Wood GW: Localization and characterization of macrophages in murine uterus. J Leukoc Biol 1985;38:255–265.
16 Matthews CJ, Adams AM, Searle RF: Detection of macrophages and the characterization of Fc receptor-bearing cells in the mouse decidua, placenta and yolk sac using the macrophage-specific monoclonal antibody F4/80. J Reprod Immunol 1985;7:315–323.
17 Oksenberg JR, Mor-Yosef S, Persitz E, et al: Antigen-presenting cells in human decidual tissue. Am J Reprod Immunol Microbiol 1986;11:82–88.
18 Kamat BR, Isaacson PG: The immunocytochemical distribution of leukocytic subpopulations in human endometrium. Am J Pathol 1987;127:66–73.
19 Bulmer JN, Morrison L, Smith JC: Expression of class II MHC gene products by macrophages in human uteroplacental tissue. Immunology 1988;63:707–714.
20 Lessin DL, Hunt JS, King CR, et al: Antigen expression by cells near the maternal-fetal interface. Am J Reprod Immunol Microbiol 1988;16:1–7.
21 Dorman PJ, Searle RF: Alloantigen presenting capacity of human decidual tissue. J Reprod Immunol 1988;13:101–112.
22 De M, Choudhuri R, Wood GW: Determination of the number and distribution of macrophages, lymphocytes, and granulocytes in the mouse uterus from mating through implantation. J Leukoc Biol 1991;50:252–262.
23 Searle RF, Wren AM: Antigen presenting capacity of human decidua: No evidence for human decidual antigen presenting cell mediated immunoregulation. J Reprod Immunol 1992;21:211–221.
24 Mizuno M, Aoki K, Kimbara T: Functions of macrophages in human decidual tissue in early pregnancy. Am J Reprod Immunol 1994;31:180–188.
25 Olivares EG, Montes MJ, Oliver C, et al: Cultured human decidual stromal cells express B7–1 (CD80) and B7–2 (CD86) and stimulate allogeneic T cells. Biol Reprod 1997;57:609–615.

26 Kammerer U, Schoppet M, McLellan AD, et al: Human decidua contains potent immunostimulatory CD83(+) dendritic cells. Am J Pathol 2000;157:159–169.
27 Soilleux EJ, Morris LS, Lee B, et al: Placental expression of DC-SIGN may mediate intrauterine vertical transmission of HIV. J Pathol 2001;195:586–592.
28 Kammerer U, Eggert AO, Kapp M, et al: Unique appearance of proliferating antigen-presenting cells expressing DC-SIGN (CD209) in the decidua of early human pregnancy. Am J Pathol 2003; 162:887–896.
29 Gardner L, Moffett A: Dendritic cells in the human decidua. Biol Reprod 2003;69:1438–1446.
30 Miyazaki S, Tsuda H, Saki M, et al: Predominance of TH2-promoting dendritic cells in early human pregnancy decidua. J Leukoc Biol 2003;74:514–522.
31 Blois SM, Alba Soto CD, Tometten M, Klapp B, Margni RA, Arck PC: Lineage, maturity, and phenotype of uterine murine dendritic cells throughout gestation indicate a protective role in maintaining pregnancy. Biol Reprod 2004;70:1018–1023.
32 Slukvin II, Breburda EE, Golos TG: Dynamic changes in primate endometrial leukocyte populations: Differential distribution of macrophages and natural killer cells at the rhesus monkey implantation site and in early pregnancy. Placenta 2004;25:297–307.
33 Lagadari M, Blois S, Margni R, Miranda S: Analysis of macrophage presence in murine placenta: Influence of age and parity status. Am J Reprod Immunol 2004;51:49–55.
34 Askelund K, Liddell HS, Zanderigo AM, et al: CD83+ dendritic cells in the decidua of women with recurrent miscarriage and normal pregnancy. Placenta 2004;25:140–145.
35 Lutz MB, Schuler G: Immature, semi-mature and fully mature dendritic cells: Which signals induce tolerance or immunity? Trends Immunol 2002;23:445–449.

Dr. Ulrike Kämmerer
Forschungslabor, Universitäts-Frauenklinik, Josef-Schneider Strasse 4
DE–97080 Würzburg (Germany), Tel. +49 931 20125293
Fax +49 931 20125406, E-Mail frak057@mail.uni-wuerzburg.de

Markert UR (ed): Immunology of Pregnancy.
Chem Immunol Allergy. Basel, Karger, 2005, vol 89, pp 105–117

Regulation of Leukocyte Recruitment to the Murine Maternal/Fetal Interface

Uta Fernekorn, Andrea Kruse

Institute of Immunology and Transfusion Medicine,
University of Lübeck, Lübeck, Germany

Abstract

Controlled immune cell access to the pregnant uterus may be one of the mechanisms involved in maternal tolerance leading to the presence of a selected population of immune cells at the maternal/fetal interface. The molecular determinants responsible for coordinating recruitment of leukocytes include the cellular adhesion molecules and members of the chemokine superfamily. During the critical period of initial placenta development in the mouse an elegantly orchestrated progression of leukocyte homing events in the decidua basalis has been described. Moreover, the maternal/fetal interface displays an unparalleled compartmentalization of microdomains associated with highly differentiated vessels expressing vascular addressins in nonoverlapping patterns. These expression patterns are functionally correlated with the distinct localization of uterine NK cells, monocyte-like cells and neutrophils. Switches in vascular specificity and the partial loss of microenvironmental specialization during the second half of mouse development have been shown to parallel dramatic changes in the populations of leukocytes recruited to the maternal/fetal interface. Recently, complex expression patterns of chemokines and their receptors were described in the human pregnant uterus suggesting that along with adhesion molecules these determinants are critical for leukocyte trafficking to the pregnant uterus.

Introduction

During the process of hemochorial placenta formation (as in rodents and primates), the genetically distinct fetal trophoblast is invading the maternal decidua and comes into intimate contact with maternal immune cells. In normal pregnancy, however, the maternal immune system fails to react to the fetus or the placenta as an allogeneic graft. Indeed those specialized leukocytes that are allowed access to the decidua are hypothesized to control trophoblast development and invasion, to function in angiogenesis and to regulate local immunity [1, 2].

Analysis of the types of immune cells that are present at the maternal/fetal interface has shown that, in both mouse and man, the predominant population represents phenotypically unusual uterine NK (uNK) cells. In rodents these unique cells increase in the mesometrial decidua just after implantation and accumulate a few days later in the mesometrial triangle between layers of the circular smooth muscle. At midterm uNK cells reach their maximal accumulation, infiltrating the whole decidua basalis and are seen in close contact with the invading trophoblast. Their numbers decline in the second half of pregnancy and only few remain in the term pregnant uterus. The fate of these cells remains uncertain. However, there is evidence that beginning at day 12 of gestation uNK cells undergo progressive nuclear fragmentation [3, 4]. Several observations suggest that uNK cells play an important role in reproduction, including regulation of trophoblast invasion and development, but a protective role against placental infections has also been proposed [5–8]. Recently, it has been shown that uNK cells are a major source of IFN-γ, which modifies the expression of genes in the uterine vasculature and stroma, initiating vessel instability and facilitating pregnancy-induced remodeling of decidual arteries [9, 10]. Cells of the myeloid lineage are also present and thought to participate in regulating many aspects of the local immune environment and of maternal/fetal tolerance. Macrophages, for example, are a major cell type in the maternal compartment of the uteroplacental unit. The production of a broad repertoire of cytokines and bioactive lipids suggests that these cells perform specific pregnancy-associated tasks [11, 12]. Recently, dendritic cells (mainly of the myeloid lineage) have been described to be present at the maternal/fetal interface in humans and mice. Several observations propose that these cells may silence T cell-dependent immune responses to trophoblast, but may also be involved in activation of uNK cells [13–15]. Neutrophils are located near the placenta where they might phagocytose cellular debris from decidual cells killed by invading trophoblast [16]. T cells, which are typical of the adaptive immune system, are rare, especially early on. Their proportion, however, increases with gestational age, followed by a decline in the term pregnant uterus. The production of a complex network of cytokines, however, suggests that T cells (together with other leukocyte subsets) could play a role on embryo development, implantation and on maternal tolerance towards the fetus [17–19].

Taken together, the decidua in pregnancy is a highly complex tissue containing unique, highly specialized leukocyte subpopulations for each stage of gestation that may play a critical role in determining the nature of local immune responses at the maternal/fetal interface. The specificity of decidual leukocyte composition during the course of pregnancy is controlled at the level of cell trafficking. This has been demonstrated in the mouse, where microdomains of differentially expressed cellular adhesion molecules involved in leukocyte recruitment have been identified at the maternal/fetal interface, especially during the critical period of initial placenta development. Switches in vascular specificity and the partial loss of microenvironmental specialization during the second half of mouse development have been shown to parallel dramatic changes in the populations of leukocytes recruited to the maternal/fetal interface [20, 21]. This review will focus on the importance of selective leukocyte trafficking to the pregnant uterus in the mouse. For a better understanding of the mechanisms and molecular determinants involved, the following section should provide a general perspective on the mechanisms of leukocyte-endothelial cell recognition which are known to play an important role in regulating the nature of immune responses in different tissues throughout the body.

The Mechanisms of Leukocyte Extravasation

Leukocyte extravasation is viewed as an active, multistep process involving initial cell-cell contact (tethering), rolling, activation through G protein-linked chemoattractant receptors, firm integrin-mediated adhesion and diapedesis. The molecular determinants responsible for coordinating recruitment and extravasation of leukocytes include the cellular adhesion molecules and members of the chemokine superfamily.

Tethering and rolling are usually mediated by the selectins and their carbohydrate ligands, but also by low-affinity α4 integrins (albeit less efficiently than selectins). Selectins consist of three members: leukocyte (L), platelet (P) and endothelial (E) selectin. They recognize distinct if overlapping sets of carbohydrate ligands, which can display considerable specificity for particular selectins at the cellular as well as the molecular level. To stop rolling leukocytes must engage secondary adhesion molecules which all belong to the integrin family. Integrins involved in leukocyte-endothelial interaction are α4 (α4β1, α4β7) and β2 (LFA-1, Mac-1) integrins which interact with members of the immunoglobulin family of adhesion molecules, mucosal addressin cell adhesion molecule-1 (MAdCAM-1), vascular cell adhesion molecule-1 (VCAM-1) and intercellular adhesion molecules (ICAMs). On most circulating and resting leukocytes, integrins are expressed in a low affinity state. To mediate leukocyte arrest and firm adhesion, integrins must become functionally upregulated. Rolling brings leukocytes into contact with the endothelium where they can sample the surface for chemoattractants that act through G protein-coupled receptors. Chemokine-induced signalling triggers rapid and dramatic changes in the adhesive function of preexisting cell surface integrins. In the presence of appropriate chemoattractant signals, activation-dependent stable arrest is followed by the final step in extravasation, called diapedesis. In this process leukocytes subsequently migrate across the endothelium to the underlying tissue parenchyma and then to distinct microenvironmental sites. These steps are also guided by adhesion molecules and multiple chemoattractant signals [reviewed in 22–26].

These considerations merely serve to emphasize the general point that complex molecular mechanisms operate coordinately to regulate local leukocyte trafficking and these mechanisms thereby play a critical role in determining the nature of local immune responses based both on the tissue involved and the nature of the physiological insult.

Leukocyte-Vascular Homing Interactions at the Maternal/Fetal Interface during the Critical Period of Initial Placenta Development

After implantation the pregnant uterus undergoes a radical transformation in structure. Uterine stromal cells proliferate and differentiate (the decidual response) producing a massive thickened uterine wall. New blood vessels develop within the decidua and existing vessels dilate. During the period of initial placenta development (day 8–10 of murine gestation) three histologically defined zones can be identified within the maternal tissue of the pregnant mouse uterus: the central decidua basalis, the vascular zone (a region of sinusoidal vessels within the decidua basalis) and the decidua capsularis (fig. 1). This time appears to be an immunologically critical period, characterized by a striking influx of maternal immune cells to the maternal/fetal interface [27]. As demonstrated in the mouse, the major infiltrating leukocyte types (neutrophils, monocyte-like cells and uNK cells) are compartmentalized into discrete, well-defined domains within the decidua basalis. The degree of separation of microenvironments is dramatic, and reminiscent of the organized architecture thought to play a significant role in regulating immune responses at the tissue level in lymphoid tissues. Moreover, each of these specialized microenvironments is associated with unique, nonoverlapping patterns of vascular adhesion receptor expression involved in leukocyte recruitment (fig. 1) [20, 21].

In the mouse an almost linear array of E-selectin has been described in the outer region of the trophoblast adjacent to the decidua basalis [20, 21]. E-selectin plays an important role in leukocyte contact and rolling in certain inflammatory models [28, 29]. In the pregnant uterus E-selectin activity is associated with maternal blood spaces containing luminally bound neutrophils and it is likely to be important in neutrophil recruitment to areas of enzymatic

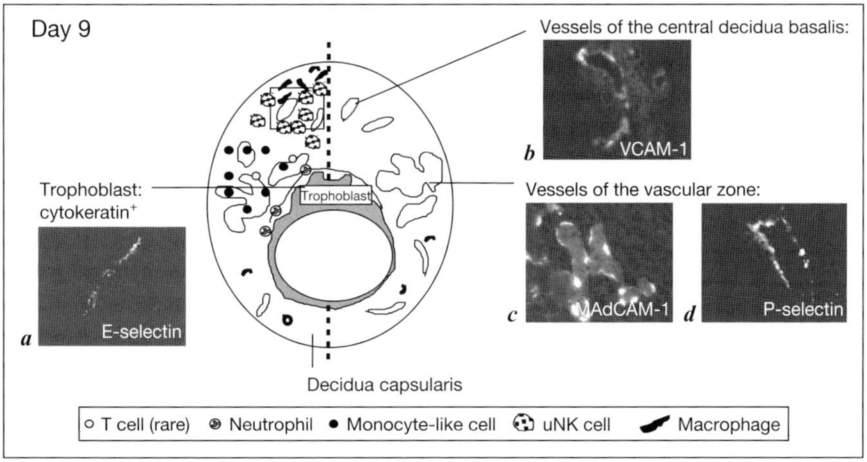

Fig. 1. Organization of day 9 pregnant mouse uterus with schematic summary of infiltrating leukocytes, distribution patterns and immunofluorescence stainings of vascular adhesion molecules. Neutrophils are limited to the leading edge of the invading trophoblast, where an almost linear array of maternal blood spaces display the neutrophil ligand E-selectin (***a***). α4β1 integrin+ uNK cells are positioned in the central decidua basalis around vessels prominently expressing the α4β1 ligand VCAM-1 (***b***). Monocyte-like cells expressing α4β7 integrin are localized in the maternal blood vessels of the vascular zone, which display the unusual combination of the α4β7 ligand MAdCAM-1 (***c***) and P-selectin (***d***) (partially associated with platelets). Magnification: ×100 (***a***); ×200 (***b–d***).

digestion at the leading edge of the invading trophoblast [16, 20]. Interestingly, several studies demonstrated the expression of E-selectin in proliferating endothelial cells of hemangiomas, neonatal foreskin and human placenta [30, 31]. Vascular endothelial cells of reproductive tissues exhibit a mitotic rate equal to or greater than that observed for tumor endothelial cells, and it has been suggested that E-selectin may also function in angiogenesis [30].

The dilated maternal vessels of the vascular zone selectively display the unusual combination of P-selectin (partially associated with platelets) and MAdCAM-1. The expression of ICAM-1 is low, in contrast to ICAM-2, which is uniformly highly expressed on maternal vessels in the pregnant uterus. The predominant cell population observed in these vessels as well as the surrounding tissue of the vascular zone belong to the monocyte/macrophage lineage. The majority of these cells express α4β7 integrin, the ligand for MAdCAM-1 [20, 21]. Interestingly, most circulating monocytes are α4β7 negative [32] while immature dendritic cells are known to express α4β7 integrin [13]. Whether these cells are monocytes or dendritic-like cells is still unknown. T and B cells are rare or even absent at this time of gestation. In the context of current multistep models of leukocyte homing, the unusual coexpression of vascular P-selectin and MAdCAM-1 in the pregnant mouse uterus may provide a mechanism for selecting specialized subsets of leukocytes displaying a unique combination of P-selectin binding and MAdCAM-1 binding activities (e.g. the $\alpha 4\beta 7+$ monocyte-like cells observed in the vessels and tissue of the vascular zone). Thus, either endothelial cells and/or platelet-associated P-selectin may initiate attachment of $\alpha 4\beta 7$ integrin expressing monocyte-like cells to the vascular zone vessels which then bind to vascular MAdCAM-1 via their $\alpha 4\beta 7$ integrin ligand. Recently, in vivo studies clearly demonstrated that both adhesion molecules are functional [21; unpubl. data] and support the importance of this unusual combination of vascular adhesion receptor expression for the recruitment of $\alpha 4\beta 7+$ monocyte-like cells to the maternal/fetal interface. Interestingly, Salmi et al. [33] reported an involvement of MAdCAM-1 in immune cell trafficking to the human uterus.

Vessels in the central microenvironment of the decidua basalis as well as those of the large venous channels at the base of the mesentery express high levels of VCAM-1 and ICAMs but no other vascular addressins. The VCAM-1+ vessels in the central decidua basalis are surrounded by uNK cells which express the VCAM-1 ligand $\alpha 4\beta 1$ integrin [20, 21]. Consistent with this, Burrows et al. [34] observed that human decidual NK cells located near VCAM-1+ vessels at the implantation site also express the $\alpha 4\beta 1$ integrin. Injection of $\alpha 4\beta 1+$ L1–2 cells into pregnant mice in the presence or absence of blocking monoclonal antibodies against VCAM-1 clearly demonstrated that vascular VCAM-1 in this site is functional [21]. It is, however, hard to imagine that such very large cells (up to 50 μm) [3] are involved in a normal process of leukocyte trafficking and extravasation. To address the question of the origin of uNK cells, it is well established in both rodents and humans that uNK cells are unable to self-renew within the uterus and early reports suggested local decidual differentiation of uNK cells from bone marrow-derived small lymphocytic precursors [35, 36]. Recently, the group of Croy [35] performed experiments in which thymus, bone marrow, lymph node or spleen cells were grafted from virgin or pregnant NK cell-competent donors into mated NK/uNK cell-deficient recipients. Interestingly, their results revealed that some secondary lymphoid tissues, especially the spleen, gave a higher level of reconstitution than primary lymphoid tissue, suggesting that precursors of uNK cells move into the uterus from secondary lymphoid tissues during pregnancy [35]. It has also been proposed that hormonal events from the decidualizing uterus may be involved in this process [37]. However, to date it is not clear whether endothelial VCAM-1, selectively and highly expressed by venules in the uNK cell-rich zone, may help mediate the recruitment of precursors of uNK cells.

Leukocyte-Vascular Homing Interactions at the Maternal/Fetal Interface from Midgestation to Term

At midterm the basic decidual zones described above remain almost intact. Differences to earlier stages include a stronger expression of vascular adhesion molecules and an increased influx of leukocytes (fig. 2). The increased recruitment of leukocytes to the maternal/fetal interface may result from a recognition of paternal MHC class I alloantigens, whose transcripts can initially be detected at day 9.5 postcoitus in the primary and secondary trophoblast giant cell populations [38]. One of the most striking observations at this period is the beginning of loss of microenvironmental specialization, a trend which continues to term. The dilated maternal vessels of the vascular zone display a combination of vascular adhesion receptors (P-selectin, MAdCAM-1 and VCAM-1) which may be unique to this setting [21]. Expression of endothelial VCAM-1 by vascular zone vessels at this stage of pregnancy and the appearance of $\alpha4\beta1$ integrin expressing uNK cells in the lumen of these vessels and the surrounding tissue suggest an involvement of VCAM-1 in the spreading and recruitment of these cells to other parts of the uterus. Within the vessels of the vascular zone adherent leukocytes are now predominantly neutrophils and monocytes with increased numbers of T cells [21, 39]. The mechanisms which are involved in T cell recruitment to these vessels are not clear. The exclusion of lymphocytes in the P-selectin+ MAdCAM-1+ vascular zone vessels in earlier stages suggests that it is unlikely that the recruited lymphocytes use MAdCAM-1 as vascular ligand. It has been shown that on most circulating lymphocytes (including $\alpha4\beta7$(hi) T cells, which tend to be $\alpha4\beta1$(lo) but not negative), binding to VCAM-1 is dominated by $\alpha4\beta1$, with $\alpha4\beta7$-VCAM-1 interaction being difficult to demonstrate except under artificial experimental conditions [23]. Thus, T cells expressing $\alpha4\beta1$ or even $\alpha4\beta7$ might be allowed access to the decidua at this time of gestation by binding to endothelial VCAM-1.

During the second half of pregnancy in the mouse the uterus lacks the microenvironmental compartmentalization mentioned above. The maternal vessels of the decidua basalis express vascular adhesion molecules in overlapping patterns (fig. 2). Changes in vascular adhesion receptor expression (decline of MAdCAM-1, upregulation of VCAM-1 and P-selectin), parallel dramatic alterations in recruited leukocyte subpopulations (decreased recruitment of monocyte-like cells, elevated influx of granulocytes and T lymphocytes) [21]. Increased recruitment of T cells during the second half of pregnancy was also described by Kearns and Lala [39]. The role of T cells at the maternal/fetal interface is not fully understood. According to Wegmann et al. [40], the maternal immune response in the pregnant uterus is biased to the less damaging Th2 type, as indicated by the fact that mouse fetomaternal tissues spontaneously secrete

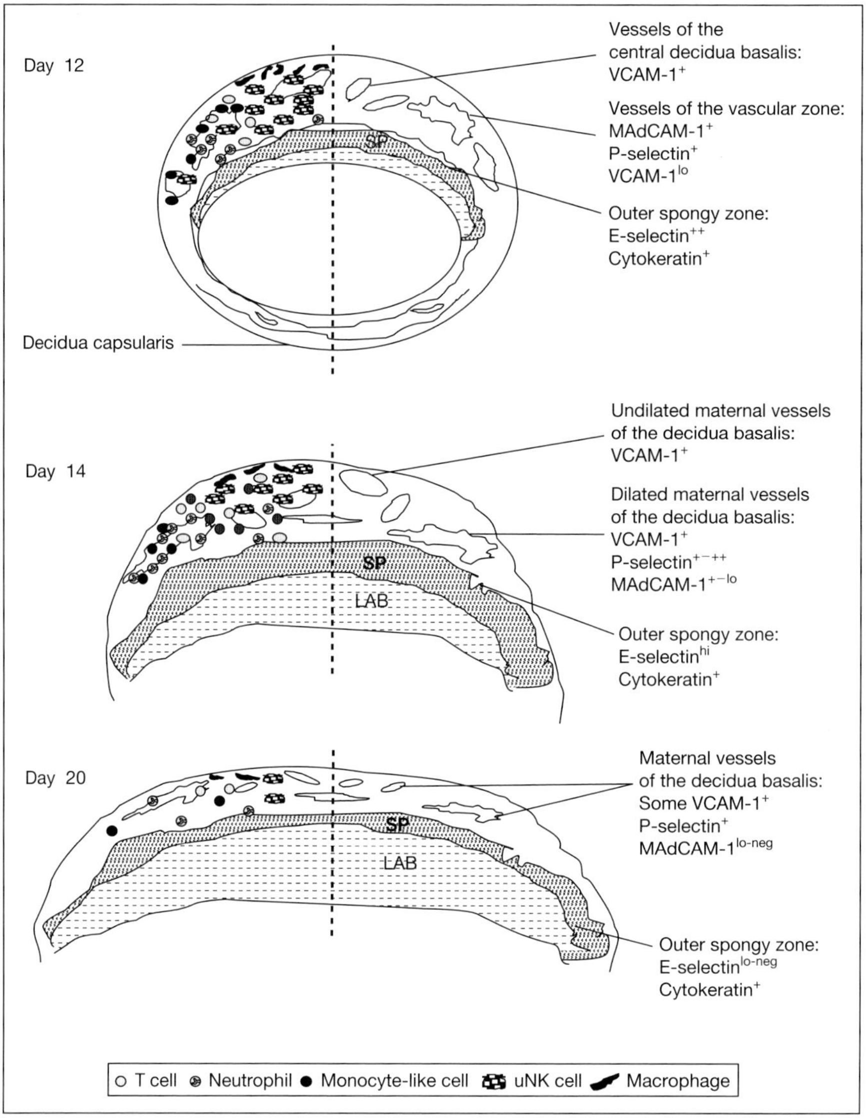

Fig. 2. Organization of the pregnant mouse uterus from gestational days 12, 14 and 20 with a schematic summary of the infiltrating leukocytes and distribution patterns of vascular adhesion molecules characteristic for each day of gestation. SP = Spongiotrophoblast (spongy zone); LAB = labyrinthine zone.

the Th2-type cytokines IL-4, IL-5 and IL-10. Other groups reported the production of both Th1 and Th2 cytokines at the maternal/fetal interface [9, 41,

42]. A recent report, however, showed that mice lacking four Th2-type cytokines can reproduce normally [43] and it has also been demonstrated in humans that regulatory indoleamine 2,3-dioxygenase-producing dendritic cells inhibited T cell proliferation [44, 45].

The term pregnant decidua in the mouse contains remarkably few maternal leukocytes (predominantly neutrophils and macrophages) (fig. 2), suggesting diminished recruitment of immune cells to the maternal/fetal interface [21]. Decreased expression of integrins, vascular addressins and vascular differentiation antigens has also been described either in the human or in the mouse placenta and decidua [27, 46, 47] suggesting that trophoblast cells and maternal endothelial cells lose their selective antigeneic characteristics when the process of placentation is complete and as the placenta dies. However, the mechanisms determining the end of pregnancy are still not well understood. Histological analysis of human myometrium during spontaneous labor at term demonstrated E-selectin expression on vascular endothelium associated with strong infiltration of neutrophils and macrophages [48]. In mouse endometrium, 1 day before parturition the macrophage population was found to be diminished by 70% whereas macrophage numbers in the myometrium remained stable [49]. Mackler et al. [49] suggested that withdrawal of these immune cells from the endometrium may eliminate a major restraint on uterine contractile activity while the macrophages residing in the myometrium may shift the balance of activity to produce inflammatory factors like IFN-γ and TNF-α that promote contraction of the uterus during labor.

Chemokines at the Maternal/Fetal Interface

Along with surface adhesion molecules chemokines play a critical role in regulating the leukocyte recruitment cascade as well as chemotaxis within tissues. To date little is known about chemokine and chemokine receptor expression and their role in leukocyte recruitment to and within the pregnant uterus. In human and mouse uteri constant expression of mRNA and protein for MCP-1, MIP-1α and RANTES have been reported during the estrous cycle. Postimplantation the expression of these chemokines increases, suggesting an involvement in leukocyte recruitment to the pregnant uterus [50–53]. Their receptors (CCR2 for MCP-1, CCR5 for MIP-1α and RANTES) are constitutively expressed on peripheral NK cells and MCP-1, MIP-1α and RANTES have been described to be potent in NK cell migration to their appropriate location in tumor-bearing and virally challenged animals [54–56]. Analysis of implantation sites of mice genetically ablated for CCR2, CCR5, MIP-1α or CCR2 and MIP-1α, however, suggests that migration and distribution of NK cells within the pregnant uterus are independent of CCR2, CCR5 and MIP-1α [51]. Recently challenging studies were performed by Red-Horse et al. [52] investigating chemokine ligand and receptor expression in the human pregnant uterus. They found a widespread expression of chemokine mRNA in the decidual stroma and specific expression patterns in decidual leukocytes and cytotrophoblast cells. Importantly, the receptors for these chemokines could be detected on decidual leukocytes. For example, chemokine receptor characteristic of NK cells, T cells and monocytes were abundant (e.g. CX3CR1, CXCR3, CCR1, CCR2, CCR5, and CCR7), as were their ligands within the decidua (fractalkine, IP-10, MIP-1α, MCP-1, HCC-1 and SLC). Several of the chemokines shared identical expression patterns at the maternal/fetal interface and some of the molecules expressed in similar locations share the same receptors suggesting overlapping functions. The chemokines seem not only to be involved in leukocyte recruitment like SLC and SDF-1 observed in the lumen of uterine vessels, but also in cell migration within the uterine tissue. Red-Horse et al. [52] suggested a possible combination of factors acting on the migration of decidual leukocytes, like SLC/CCR7 for extravasation, HCC-1/CCR1 for moving within the decidual stroma and IP-10/CXCR3 to cluster the cells near glands. Middleton et al. [57] demonstrated that endothelial cells in general transport chemokines from the basolateral to the luminal surface, so that it is likely that chemokines produced in the uterine tissue can also impact on leukocyte recruitment.

Taken together, the extravasation of leukocytes from the blood to the tissue of the pregnant uterus needs to be a well-controlled process to ensure the recruitment of the right cells to the correct location at the right time. The highly regulated expression of vascular addressins clearly indicates that adhesion receptor expression and, more generally, mechanisms of vascular differentiation and specialization are fundamental to this process. Recent studies in the human uterus clearly indicate that chemokines and their receptors may play a critical role in leukocyte trafficking to the maternal/fetal interface.

References

1. Tartakovsky B, Ben-Yair E: Cytokines modulate preimplantation development and pregnancy. Dev Biol 1991;146:345–352.
2. Piccinni MP: Role of immune cells in pregnancy. Autoimmunity 2003;36:1–4.
3. Bulmer D, Peel S, Stewart I: The metrial gland. Cell Differ 1987;20:77–86.
4. Delgado SR, McBey BA, Yamashiro S, Fujita J, Kiso Y, Croy BA: Accounting for the peripartum loss of granulated metrial gland cells, a natural killer population, from the pregnant uterus. J Leukoc Biol 1996;59:262–269.
5. Croy BA: Granulated metrial gland cells – interesting cells found in the pregnant uterus. Am J Reprod Immunol 1990;23:19–21.

6 Mingari MC, Ponte M, Cantono C, Moretta L: Natural killer cells in pregnancy: How do they avoid attacking fetal tissue? Immunologist 1999;7:107–111.
7 King A, Loke YW, Chaouat G: NK cells and reproduction. Immunol Today 1997;18:64–66.
8 Biassoni R, Bottino C, Millo R, Moretta L, Moretta A: Natural killer cell-mediated recognition of human trophoblast. Semin Cancer Biol 1999;9:13–18.
9 Platt JS, Hunt JS: Interferon-γ gene expression in cycling and pregnant mouse uterus: Temporal aspects and cellular localization. J Leukoc Biol 1998;6:393–400.
10 Ashkar AA, Di Santo JP, Croy BA: Interferon γ contributes to initiation of uterine vascular modification, decidual integrity, and uterine natural killer cell maturation during normal murine pregnancy. J Exp Med 2000;192:259–270.
11 Hunt JS: Cytokine networks in the uteroplacental unit: Macrophages pivotal regulatory cells. J Reprod Immunol 1989;16:1–17.
12 Hunt JS, Robertson SA: Uterine macrophages and environmental programming for pregnancy success. J Reprod Immunol 1986;32:1–25.
13 Kämmerer U, Schoppet M, McLellan AD, Kapp M, Huppertz H-I, Kampgen E, Dietl J: Human decidua contains potent immunostimulatory CD83+ dendritic cells. Am J Pathol 2000;157: 159–169.
14 Gardner L, Moffett A: Dendritic cells in the human decidua. Biol Reprod 2003;69:1438–1446.
15 Blois S, Alba Soto CD, Tometten M, Klapp BF, Margni RA, Arck PC: Lineage, maturity and phenotype of uterine murine dendritic cells throughout gestation indicate a protective role in maintaining pregnancy. Biol Reprod 2004;70:1020–1034.
16 Parr EL, Young LH, Parr MB, Young JD: Granulated metrial gland cells of the pregnant mouse uterus are natural killer-like cells that contain perforin and serine esterases. J Immunol 1990; 145:2365–2372.
17 Mellor AL, Munn DH: Immunology at the maternal-fetal interface: Lessons for T cell tolerance and suppression. Annu Rev Immunol 2000;18:367–391.
18 Chaouat G, Zourbas S, Ostojic S, Lappree-Delage G, Dubanchet S, Ledee N, Martal J: A brief review of recent data on some cytokine expressions at the materno-foetal interface which might challenge the classical Th1/Th2 dichotomy. J Reprod Immunol 2002;53:241–256.
19 Aluvihare VR, Kallikourdis M, Betz AG: Regulatory T cells mediate maternal tolerance to the fetus. Nat Immunol 2004;5:266–271.
20 Kruse A, Merchant MJ, Hallmann R, Butcher EC: Evidence of specialized leukocyte-vascular homing interactions at the maternal/fetal interface. Eur J Immunol 1999;29:1116–1126.
21 Kruse A, Martens N, Fernekorn U, Hallmann R, Butcher EC: Alterations in the expression of homing-associated molecules at the maternal/fetal interface during the course of pregnancy. Biol Reprod 2002;66:333–345.
22 Springer TA: Traffic signals on endothelium for lymphocyte recirculation and leukocyte emigration. Annu Rev Physiol 1995;57:827–872.
23 Butcher EC, Williams M, Youngman K, Rott LS, Briskin MJ: Lymphocyte trafficking and regional immunity. Adv Immunol 1999;72:209–253.
24 Von Andrian UH, Mackay CR: T-cell function and migration. Two sides of the same coin. N Engl J Med 2000;343:1020–1034.
25 Johnston B, Butcher EC: Chemokines in rapid leukocyte adhesion triggering and migration. Semin Immunol 2002;14:83–92.
26 Campbell DJ, Kim CH, Butcher EC: Chemokines in the systemic organization of immunity. Immunol Rev 2003;195:58–71.
27 Cross JC, Werb Z, Fisher SJ: Implantation and the placenta: Key pieces of the development puzzle. Science 1994;266:1508–1518.
28 Abbassi O, Kishimoto TK, McIntire LV, Anderson DC, Smith CW: E-selectin supports neutrophil rolling in vitro under conditions of flow. J Clin Invest 1993;92:2710–2730.
29 Olofsson AM, Arfors KE, Ramezani L, Wolitzky BA, Butcher EC, von Andrian UH: E-selectin mediates leukocyte rolling in interleukin-1 treated rabbit mesentery venules. Blood 1994;84: 2749–2758.
30 Kräling BM, Razon MJ, Boon LM, Zurakowski D, Seachord C, Darveau RP, Mulliken JB, Corless CL, Bischoff J: E-selectin is present in proliferating endothelial cells in human hemangiomas. Am J Pathol 1996;148:1181–1191.

31 Ruck P, Marzusch K, Kaiserling E, Horny H-P, Dietl J, Geiselhart A, Handgretinger R, Redman CWG: Distribution of cell adhesion molecules in decidua of early human pregnancy. An immunohistochemical study. Lab Invest 1994;71:94–101.
32 Tiisala S, Paavonen T, Renkonen R: AlphaE beta7 and alpha4 beta7 integrins associated with intraepithelial and mucosal homing are expressed on macrophages. Eur J Immunol 1995; 25:411–417.
33 Salmi M, Alanen K, Grenman S, Briskin M, Butcher EC, Jalkanen S: Immune cell trafficking in uterus and early life is dominated by the mucosal addressin MAdCAM-1 in humans. Gastroenterology 2001;121:853–864.
34 Burrows TD, King A, Loke YW: Expression of adhesion molecules by human decidual large granular lymphocytes. Cell Immunol 1993;147:81–94.
35 Chantakru S, Miller C, Roach LE, Kuziel WA, Maeda N, Wang WC, Evans SS, Croy BA: Contributions from self-renewal and trafficking to the uterine NK cell population of early pregnancy. J Immunol 2002;168:22–28.
36 Peel S, Stewart I, Bulmer D: Experimental evidence for the bone marrow origin of granulated metrial gland cells of the mouse uterus. Cell Tissue Res 1983;233:647–656.
37 Chantakru S, Wang WC, van den Heuvel M, Bashar S, Simpson A, Chen Q, Croy BA, Evans SS: Coordinate regulation of lymphocyte-endothelial interactions by pregnancy-associated hormones. J Immunol 2003;171:4011–4019.
38 Jaffe L, Robertson EJ, Bikoff EK: Distinct patterns of expression of MHC class I and β2 microglobulin transcripts at early stages of mouse development. J Immunol 1991;147:2740–2750.
39 Kearns M, Lala PK: Characterization of hematogenous cellular constituents of the murine decidua: A surface marker study. J Reprod Immunol 1985;8:213–234.
40 Wegmann TG, Lin H, Guilbert L, Mosmann TR: Bidirectional cytokine interactions in the maternal-fetal relationship: Is successful pregnancy a T_H2 phenomenon? Immunol Today 1993; 14:353–356.
41 Librach C, Feigenbaum S, Bass K, Cui T, Verastas N, Sadovsky Y, Quigley J, French D, Fisher S: Interleukin-1 beta regulates human cytotrophoblast metalloproteinase activity and invasion in vitro. J Biol Chem 1994;269:17125–17131.
42 Roth I, Corry D, Locksley R, Abrams J, Litton M, Fisher S: Human placental cytotrophoblasts produce the immunosuppressive cytokine IL-10. J Exp Med 1996;184:539–548.
43 Fallon PG, Jolin HE, Smith P, Emson CL, Townsend MJ, Fallon R, Smith P, McKenzie AN: IL-4 induces characteristic Th2 responses even in the combined absence of IL-5, IL-9, and IL-13. Immunity 2002;17:7–17.
44 Mellor AL, Munn DH: Tryptophan catabolism and T cell tolerance: Immunosuppression by starvation. Immunol Today 1999;20:469–473.
45 Finger EB, Bluestone JA: When ligand becomes receptor – tolerance via B7 signalling on DCs. Nat Immunol 2002;2:1056–1057.
46 Damsky CH, Librach C, Lim KH, Fitzgerald ML, McMaster MT, Janatpour M, Zhou Y, Logan SK, Fisher SJ: Integrin switching regulates normal trophoblast invasion. Development 1994;120: 3657–3666.
47 Kruse A, Hallmann R, Butcher EC: Specialized patterns of vascular differentiation antigens in the pregnant mouse uterus and the placenta. Biol Reprod 1999;61:1393–1401.
48 Thomson AJ, Telfer JF, Young A, Campbell S, Stewart CJR, Cameron IT, Greer IA, Norman JE: Leukocytes infiltrate the myometrium during human parturition: Further evidence that labour is an inflammatory process. Hum Reprod 1999;14:229–236.
49 Mackler AM, Green LM, McMillan PJ, Yellon SM: Distribution and activation of uterine mononuclear phagocytes in peripartum endometrium and myometrium of the mouse. Biol Reprod 2000; 62:1193–1200.
50 Hornung D, Ryan I, Chao V, Vigne J, Schriock E, Taylor R: Immunolocalization and regulation of the chemokine RANTES in human endometrial and endometriosis tissues and cells. J Clin Endocrinol Metab 1997;82:1621–1628.
51 Chantakru S, Kuziel WA, Maeda N, Croy BA: A study on the density and distribution of uterine natural killer cells at mid pregnancy in mice genetically-ablated for CCR2, CCR5 and the CCR5 receptor ligand, MIP-1α. J Reprod Immunol 2001;49:33–47.

52 Red-Horse K, Drake PM, Gunn MD, Fisher SJ: Chemokine ligand and receptor expression in the pregnant uterus. Reciprocal patterns in complementary cell subsets suggest functional roles. Am J Pathol 2001;159:2199–2213.
53 Ramhorst RE, Garcia VE, Corigliano A, Rabinovich GA, Fainboim L: Identification of RANTES as a novel immunomodulator of the maternal allogeneic response. Clin Immunol 2004;110:71–80.
54 Polentarutti N, Allavena O, Bianchi G, Giardina G, Basaile A, Sozzani S, Mantovani A, Introna M: IL-2-regulated expression of the monocyte chemotactic protein-1 receptor (CCR2) in human NK cells. J Immunol 1997;158:2689–2694.
55 Neito M, Navaro F, Perz-Villar JJ, del Pozo MA, Gonzalez-Amaro R, Mellado M, Frade JMR, Martinez A, Lopez-Botet M, Sanchez-Madrid F: Roles of chemokines and receptor polarization in NK-target cell interactions. J Immunol 1998;161:3330–3339.
56 Cook DN, Beck MA, Coffman TM, Kirby SL, Sheridan JF, Pragnell IB, Smithies O: Requirement of MIP-1α for an inflammatory response to virus infection. Science 1995;269:1583–1585.
57 Middleton J, Neil S, Wintle J, Clark-Lewis I, Moore H, Lam C, Auer M, Hub E, Rot A: Transcytosis and surface presentation of IL-8 by venular endothelial cells. Cell 1997;91:385–395.

Andrea Kruse
Institute of Immunology and Transfusion Medicine
University of Lübeck, School of Medicine, Ratzeburger Allee 160
DE–23538 Lübeck (Germany), Tel. +49 451 5003462
Fax +49 451 5002857, E-Mail Kruse@immu.mu-luebeck.de

Market UR (ed): Immunology of Pregnancy.
Chem Immunol Allergy. Basel, Karger, 2005, vol 89, pp 118–125

Progesterone-Dependent Immunomodulation

J. Szekeres-Bartho, B. Polgar, N. Kozma, E. Miko, G. Par, L. Szereday, A. Barakonyi, T. Palkovics, O. Papp, P. Varga

Department of Medical Microbiology and Immunology, Pecs University, Medical School, Reproductive and Tumor Immunology Research Group of the Hungarian Academy of Sciences, Pecs, Hungary

Abstract

The biological effects of progesterone are mediated by a 34-kDa protein named the progesterone-induced blocking factor (PIBF). PIBF, synthesized by lymphocytes of healthy pregnant women in the presence of progesterone, inhibits arachidonic acid release as well as NK activity, and modifies the cytokine balance. Within the cell the full-length PIBF is associated with the centrosome, while secretion of shorter forms is induced by activation of the cell. PIBF induces nuclear translocation of STAT6 as well as PKC phosphorylation and exerts a negative effect on STAT4 phosphorylation. The concentration of PIBF in pregnancy urine is related to the positive or negative outcome of pregnancy; furthermore, premature pregnancy termination is predictable by lower than normal pregnancy PIBF values. In vivo data suggest the biological importance of the above findings. Treatment of pregnant Balb/c mice with the antiprogesterone RU 486 results in an increased resorption rate, which is associated with the inability of spleen cells to produce PIBF. High resorption rates induced by progesterone receptor block as well as those due to high NK activity are corrected by simultaneous PIBF treatment.

Progesterone-Induced Blocking Factor Mediates the Immunological Effects of Progesterone

Beside its well-known endocrine effects, progesterone is endowed with immunomodulatory properties, which contribute to its pregnancy-protective role. High concentrations of progesterone prolong the survival of xenogenic and allogenic grafts [1, 2], and the hormone affects various phases of the immune response in vitro [3–5].

NK activity of lymphocytes of healthy pregnant women can be suppressed by a relatively low (100–400 n*M*) concentration of progesterone, whereas 100 times higher concentrations are required for reducing the natural cytotoxic activity of nonpregnancy lymphocytes [6] and this effect is inhibited by equimolar concentrations of RU 486 (a blocker of progesterone and glucocorticoid receptors) [7].

The biological effects of progesterone are mediated by a 34-kDa protein, named the progesterone-induced blocking factor (PIBF). PIBF, synthesized by lymphocytes of healthy pregnant women in the presence of progesterone [8, 9], inhibits arachidonic acid release by acting directly on the phophopase A2 enzyme [10] as well as NK activity and modifies the cytokine balance [11]. Through the above mechanisms PIBF exerts an antiabortive effect [12–14].

Molecular Structure of PIBF

The PIBF cDNA encodes a protein of 757-amino acid residues with an 89-kDa predicted molecular mass, which shows no significant amino acid sequence homology with any of the known proteins [15].

The full-length PIBF is associated with the centrosome, while secretion of shorter forms, among others; the previously described secreted 34-kDa protein is induced by activation of the cell. The 48-kDa N-terminal part of PIBF is biologically active, and the region responsible for modulating NK activity is encoded by exons 2–4 [15]. These data suggest that PIBF might act both as a transcription factor and as a cytokine, via binding to receptors.

Biological Effects of PIBF

PIBF affects arachidonic acid metabolism of lymphoid cells and the subsequent decrease in prostaglandin and/or leukotriene synthesis goes in parallel with lower cytotoxic activity [8]. IL-12 induces NK activity and there is evidence for a relationship between high NK activity and pregnancy termination both in mice [16, 17] and humans [18]. In our hands, neutralization of PIBF resulted in an increased IL-12 expression, which was corrected by treatment of the cells with phospholipase A2 inhibitor [10].

These results suggest that PIBF inhibits arachidonic acid release. The subsequent block of prostaglandin synthesis reduces IL-12 production and results in a lowered cytotoxic NK activity, which favors a normal pregnancy outcome. In line with this hypothesis, aspirin treatment starting before implantation may reduce the rate of abortion in patients suffering from recurrent miscarriages [19]. Furthermore, the frequency of postmaturity and the length of gestation were significantly increased in women who regularly took large doses of prostaglandin synthesis inhibitors [20].

Cytokine Effects and Signal Transduction

The effect of PIBF on NK activity is manifested via an altered cytokine production both in vitro and in vivo. Neutralization of endogenous PIBF in pregnancy lymphocytes by a PIBF-specific antibody results in increased NK activity, which is corrected by IL-12-neutralizing antibody [11]. PIBF inhibits IL-12 synthesis by activated lymphocytes, and recent data from our laboratory revealed an increased IL-12 production by peripheral lymphocytes of women with pathological pregnancies and high NK activity [21]. In vitro PIBF treatment of activated lymphocytes favors the production of Th2 type of cytokines [22]. Joachim et al. [23] detected reduced PIBF concentrations, together with increased resorption rates in pregnant mice that had been subjected to acoustic stress. Both PIBF levels and resorption rates were corrected by treating the animals with a retroprogesterone, and this was accompanied by a significantly increased decidual IL-4 production. These data together support the concept that the NK inhibitory action of PIBF is mediated – at least in part – by cytokines, and PIBF induces a Th2-biased cytokine production.

STAT transcription factors mediate virtually all cytokine-driven signaling, whereas protein kinase C (PKC) plays a critical role in the differentiation of T cells to the Th1 or Th2 type.

STAT6 and STAT4 specifically mediate signals that stem from IL-4 and IL-12 receptors, respectively [24]. INF-γ has been shown to be a negative regulator of STAT6-dependent transcription of target genes [25]. STAT4 is mainly phosphorylated by the IL-12-mediated signaling pathway in T cells and in NK cells by the tyrosine kinases Jak2 and Tyk2 [26, 27]. Mice lacking STAT4 clearly demonstrated that STAT4 is necessary for the generation of Th1 cells [28, 29].

STAT6-deficient animals are unable to mount an immune response to helminthic parasites and therefore are unable to clear the parasitic infections [30]. IL-4 signaling via STAT6 appears to play role in the development of allergic asthma; it has been also observed that STAT6-deficient mice did not develop airway hyperresponsiveness after allergen sensitization like their wild-type littermates and were protected from allergic asthma [31].

The 48-kDa recombinant human PIBF as well as two smaller proteins encoded by exons 2–4 and 13–16 induce nuclear translocation of STAT6 [32].

PIBF exerts a negative effect on STAT4 phosphorylation and inhibits IL-12-induced STAT4 activation.

The PKC pathway represents a major signal transduction system that is activated following ligand stimulation of receptors by hormones, neurotransmitters, and growth factors. PKC (80-kDa proteins) play a critical role in the regulation of differentiation and proliferation in many cell types and in the response to diverse stimuli [33].

Development of naive T cells into type 1 (Th1) or type 2 (Th2) effector cells is thought to be under the control of cytokines. IL-12 and IL-4 are widely accepted to be the major factors inducing T cells to develop into type 1 or type 2 cells [34]. When IL-12 and IL-4 are present, murine and human T cell differentiation is regulated by the balance of PKC and calcium signaling within T cells [35].

It has long been known that Th2 clones show reduced calcium flux after activation compared with Th1 clones [36]. High levels of PKC activity combined with low calcium signals favor Th2 development, while predominance of calcium signaling with low PKC activity favors Th1 development [35]. Signals downstream of PKC and calcineurin directly result in preferential type 1 or type 2 cytokine gene expressions, perhaps via expression of transcription factors associated with Th2 cells [37, 38].

Phosphorylation of PKC is increased in the cytoplasmic fraction of lymphocytes treated with the 48-kDa recombinant PIBF as well as with a peptide encoded by exons 13–16. Intracellular calcium levels are not altered by PIBF treatment. High PKC activity and low intracellular calcium levels favor the development of Th2 cytokine-sensitive cells, whereas inhibition of STAT4 phosphorylation decreases the sensitivity of the cell to Th1 cytokines. These together might account for the Th2-biased immune response induced by PIBF [32].

PIBF Concentration in Pregnancy Urine Is Related to the Outcome of Pregnancy

PIBF is a secreted molecule; thus it might appear in biological fluids, and due to its small molecular weight, it is filtrated into the urine. Urinary PIBF concentrations of 86 healthy nonpregnant individuals and those from 496 pregnant women were determined by ELISA. The concentration of PIBF continuously increased until the 37th gestational week of normal pregnancies, followed by a sharp decrease after the 41st week of gestation. In pathological pregnancies urinary PIBF levels failed to increase. Samples from 86 healthy nonpregnant individuals were used for determining the threshold of nonpregnancy values. Eighty percent of women with a normal, uneventful pregnancy whereas only 10% of those whose pregnancies ended up in miscarriage, or preterm labor had higher PIBF concentrations than control threshold. The sensitivity (defined as the ability to correctly identify those who will deliver preterm) and specificity (the ability to correctly identify those who will not deliver preterm) of the test for predicting pregnancy failure are 90 and 80%, respectively. These data suggest that low PIBF values might indicate the onset of spontaneous pregnancy termination.

Women with toxemia had lower PIBF values than healthy pregnant women. Since PIBF favors a Th2 cytokine response, these women should have a relative Th1 dominance. Rein et al. [39] reported that trophoblast cells from preeclamptic women produce significantly less IL-10 in the 3rd trimester of pregnancy than those from healthy pregnant women, and an excessive Th1 activity has been associated with toxemia [40]. Several studies have shown that the clinical severity of preeclampsia is related to the severity of cytokine abnormalities [41]. PIBF concentrations in urine of toxemic women were related to the clinical symptoms. PIBF levels of women demonstrating hypertension only did not differ from those of healthy pregnant women. In contrast to this, only 33% of women with two or more symptoms had levels higher than the threshold. This is in line with earlier observations of Varga et al. [42], who could not demonstrate an increased peripheral NK activity in the group of preeclamptic patients with a single symptom (hypertension), whereas lymphocytes of preeclamptic women with at least two symptoms showed a significantly increased NK activity. PIBF inhibits NK activity both in vitro [2, 5], and the lack of PIBF results in an increased NK activity [11].

All the women bearing small-for-date babies had lower than normal PIBF values. This suggests that similar mechanisms might play a role in the development of intrauterine growth retardation. Bartha et al. [43] have shown an association between increased TNF-α levels and intrauterine growth retardation. In our hands treatment of pregnant mice with high NK activity spleen cells resulted in elevated serum and placental TNF-α levels in pregnant Balb/c mice, together with increased resorption rates. Simultaneous TNF-α administration corrected both TNF-α levels and resorption rates. In vitro data suggest that PIBF counteracts the cytotoxic action of TNF-α but does not interfere with its production [44].

In general, the concentration of PIBF is related to the positive or negative outcome of pregnancy; furthermore, premature pregnancy termination is predictable by lower than normal pregnancy PIBF values.

PIBF Exerts an Antiabortive Effect in Mice

In vivo data suggest the biological importance of the above findings. Treatment of pregnant Balb/c mice with the antiprogesterone RU 486 results in an increased resorption rate, which is associated with the inability of spleen cells to produce PIBF. High resorption rates induced by progesterone receptor block as well as those due to high NK activity are corrected by simultaneous PIBF treatment [13, 14].

Neutralization of endogenous PIBF by a PIBF-specific antibody terminates pregnancy in mice [11]. Depletion of NK activity with anti-NK antibodies counteracts the above effects [45]. Both anti-PIBF treatment and that with progesterone receptor blocker result in increased splenic NK activity, together with reduced IL-10 and an increased IFN-γ? production of the spleen cells.

Based on these data we suggest that the immunological pregnancy-protective effects of progesterone are manifested via the following mechanism: in the presence of progesterone activated pregnancy lymphocytes synthesize a mediator (PIBF), which, by interfering with arachidonic acid metabolism and by inducing a Th2-biased immune response, allows pregnancy to go to term.

Acknowledgment

Several authors of this manuscript are members of an European Network of Excellence, entitled "EMBIC" (Embryo Implantation Control), supported by the European Union (contract no. 512040). This work was supported by grants from the Hungarian National Research Fund (OTKA T031737), the Hungarian Ministry of Health (ETT 45/2003) and the Hungarian Academy of Sciences.

References

1 Moriyama I, Sugawa T: Progesterone facilitates implantation of xenogenic cultured cells in hamster uterus. Nat New Biol 1972;236:150–152.

2 Hansen PJ, Bazer FW, Segerson EC: Skin graft survival in the uterine lumen of ewes treated with progesterone. Am J Reprod Immunol Microbiol 1986;12:48–54.

3 Siiteri PK, Febres F, Clemens LE, Chang RJ, Gondos B, Stites DP: Progesterone and the maintenance of pregnancy: Is progesterone nature's immunosuppressant? Ann NY Acad Sci 1977; 286:384–397.

4 Staples LD, Heap RB: Studies on steroids and proteins in relation to the immunology of pregnancy in the sheep; in Crighton DB (ed): Immunological Aspects of Reproduction in Mammals. London, Butterworths, 1984, pp 195–205.

5 Stites DB, Bugbee S, Siiteri PK: Differential actions of progesterone and cortisol on lymphocyte and monocyte interaction during lymphocyte activation. Relevance to immunosuppression in pregnancy. J Reprod Immunol 1983;5:215–228.

6 Szekeres-Bartho J, Hadnagy J, Pacsa AS: The suppressive effect of progesterone on lymphocyte cytotoxicity: Unique progesterone sensitivity of pregnancy lymphocytes. J Reprod Immunol 1985; 7:121–128.

7 Szekeres-Bartho J, Philibert D, Chaouat G: Progesterone suppression of pregnancy lymphocytes is not mediated by a glucocorticoid effect. Am J Reprod Immunol 1990;23:42–43.

8 Szekeres-Bartho J, Kilar F, Falkay G, Csernus V, Torok A, Pacsa AS: Progesterone-treated lymphocytes of healthy pregnant women release a factor inhibiting cytotoxicity and prostaglandin synthesis. Am J Reprod Immunol Microbiol 1985;9:15–19.

9 Szekeres-Bartho J, Autran B, Debre P, Andreu G, Denver L, Chaouat G: Immunoregulatory effects of a suppressor factor from healthy pregnant women's lymphocytes after progesterone induction. Cell Immunol 1989;122:281–294.
10 Par G, Geli J, Kozma N, Varga P, Szekeres-Bartho J: Progesterone regulates IL12 expression in pregnancy lymphocytes by inhibiting phospholipase A2. Am J Reprod Immunol 2003;49:1–5.
11 Szekeres-Bartho J, Par G, Szereday L, Smart CY, Achacz I: Progesterone and non-specific immunological mechanisms in pregnancy. Am J Reprod Immunol 1997;38:176–180.
12 Szekeres-Bartho J, Chaouat G: Lymphocyte-derived, progesterone-induced blocking factor corrects resorption in murine abortion system. Am J Reprod Immunol 1990;23:26–28.
13 Szekeres-Bartho J, Kinsky R, Chaouat G: The effect of a progesterone induced immunologic blocking factor on NK mediated resorption. Am J Reprod Immunol 1990;24:105–107.
14 Szekeres-Bartho J, Kinsky R, Chaouat G: A progesterone-induced immunologic blocking factor corrects high resorption rates in mice treated with antiprogesterone. Am J Obstet Gynecol 1990; 163:220–223.
15 Polgar B, Kispal G, Lachmann M, Paar C, Nagy E, Csere P, Miko E, Szereday L, Varga P, Szekeres-Bartho J: Molecular cloning and immunological characterization of a novel cDNA coding for PIBF. J Immunol 2003;171:5956–5963.
16 Gendron R, Baines M: Infiltrating decidual natural killer cells are associated with spontaneous abortions in mice. Cell Immunol 1988;113:261–268.
17 De Fougerolles R, Baines M: Modulation of natural killer activity influences resorption rates in CBA × DBA/2 matings. J Reprod Immunol 1987;11:147–153.
18 Aoki K, Kajiura S, Matsumoto Y, Ogasawara M, Okada S, Yagami Y, Gleicher N: Preconceptional natural-killer-cell activity as a predictor of miscarriage. Lancet 1995;345:1340–1342.
19 Kwak JYH, Gilman-Sachs A, Beaman KD, Beer AE: Reproductive outcome in women with recurrent spontaneous abortions of alloimmune and autoimmune causes: Preconception versus postconception treatment. Am J Obstet Gynecol 1992;166:1787–1795.
20 Lewis RB, Schulam JD: Influence of acetylsalicylic acid: An inhibitor of prostaglandin synthesis on the duration of human gestation and labour. Lancet 1973;ii:1159–1161.
21 Szereday L, Varga P, Szekeres-Bartho J: Cytokine production in pregnancy. Am J Reprod Immunol 1997;38:418–421.
22 Szekeres-Bartho J, Wegmann TG: A progesterone-dependent immunomodulatory protein alters the Th1/Th2 balance. J Reprod Immunol 1996;31:81–95.
23 Joachim R, Zenclussen AC, Polgar B, Douglas AJ, Fest S, Knackstedt M, Klapp BF, Arck PC: The progesterone derivative dydrogesterone abrogates murine stress-triggered abortion by inducing a Th2 biased local immune response. Steroids 2003;68:931–940.
24 Nelms K, Keegan AD, Zamorano J, Ryan JJ, Paul WE: The IL-4 receptor signaling mechanisms and biologic functions. Annu Rev Immunol 1999;17:701–738.
25 Venkataraman C, Leung S, Salvekar A, Mano H, Schindler U: Repression of IL-4 induced gene expression by INF-gamma requires STAT-1 activation. J Immunol 1999;162:4053–4061.
26 Bacon CH, Petricoin EF 3rd, Ortaldo JR, Rees RC, Lamer AC, Johnston JA, O'Shea JJ: IL-12 induces tyrosine phosphorylation and activation of STAT4 in human lymphocytes. Proc Natl Acad Sci USA 1995;92:7307–7311.
27 Wang KS, Ritz J, Frank DA: IL-2 induces STAT4 activation in primary NK cells and NK cell lines but not in T cells. J Immunol 1999;162:299–304.
28 Kaplan MH, Sun YL, Hoey T, Grusby MJ: Impaired IL-12 responses and enhanced development of Th2 cells in STAT4-deficient mice. Nature 1996;382:174–177.
29 Thierfelder WE, van Deursen JM, Yamamoto K, Tripp RA, Sarawar SR, Carson RT, Sangster MY, Avignali DA, Doherty PC, Kaplan GC, Grosveld GC, Ihle JN: Requirement for Stat4 in interleukin-12-mediated responses of natural killer and T cells. Nature 1996;382:171–174.
30 Whitfield MH, Boros JR, Grusby MJ: Th2 cells are required for *Schistosoma mansoni* egg-induced granulomatous response. J Immunol 1998;160:1850–1856.
31 Kuperman D, Schofield B, Wills-Karp M, Grusby MJ: Signal transducer and activation of transcription factor 6 (STAT6) deficient mice and protected from antigen-induced airway hyperresponsiveness and mucus production. J Exp Med 1998;187:939–948.

32 Kozma N, Pár G, Gajdos G, Keszei M, Szalai C, Falus A, Kiss K, Szeberényi J, Szekeres-Barthó J: Signal transduction pathways mediating the effects of progesterone induced blocking factor (PIBF). Submitted.
33 Newton AC: Regulation of protein kinase C. Curr Opin Cell Biol 1997;9:161.
34 Bradley LM, Yoshimoto K, Swain SL: The cytokines IL-4, INF-gamma and IL-12 regulate the development of subsets of memory effector helper T cells in vitro. J Immunol 1995;155:1713.
35 Noble A, Truman JP, Vyas B, Vukmanovic-Stejk M, Hirst WJ, Kemeny DM: The balance of protein kinase C and calcium signaling directs T cell subset development. J Immunol 2000;164:1807.
36 Gajewski TF, Schell SR, Fitch FW: Evidence implicating utilization of different T cell receptor-associated signaling pathways by Th1 and Th2 clones. J Immunol 1990;144:4110.
37 Miner K, Croft M: Generation, persistence and modulation of Th0 effector cells: Role of autocrine IL-4 and INFγ. J Immunol 1998;160:5280.
38 Ho IC, Lo D, Glimcher LH: C-maf promotes T helper cell type 2 (Th2) and attenuates Th1 differentiation by both interleukin-4-dependent and -independent mechanism. J Exp Med 1998; 188:1859.
39 Rein DT, Breidenbach M, Honscheid B, Friebe-Hoffmann U, Engel H, Gohring UJ, Uekermann L, Kurbacher CM, Schondorf T: Preeclamptic women are deficient of interleukin-10 as assessed by cytokine release of trophoblast cells in vitro. Cytokine 2003;23:119–125.
40 Wilczynski JR, Tchorzewski H, Banasik M, Glowacka E, Wieczorek A, Lewkowicz P, Malinowski A, Szpakowski M, Wilczynski J: Lymphocyte subset distribution and cytokine secretion in third trimester decidua in normal pregnancy and preeclampsia. Eur J Obstet Gynecol Reprod Biol 2003; 109:8–15.
41 Madazli R, Aydin S, Uludag S, Vildan O, Tolun N: Maternal plasma levels of cytokines in normal and preeclamptic pregnancies and their relationship with diastolic blood pressure and fibronectin levels. Acta Obstet Gynecol Scand 2003;82:797–802.
42 Varga P, Gunther W, Bolte A, Szekeres-Bartho J: Natural lymphocyte cytotoxicity of women with different symptoms of toxaemia. Eur J Obstet Gynecol Reprod Biol 1991;16:133–137.
43 Bartha JL, Romero-Carmona R, Comino-Delgado R: Inflammatory cytokines in intrauterine growth retardation. Acta Obstet Gynecol Scand 2003;82:1099–1102.
44 Szekeres-Bartho J, Kinsky R, Kapovic M, Chaouat G, Varga P, Csiszar T: The role of immunoendocrine mechanisms in pregnancy termination; in Dondero F, Johnson PM (eds): Reproductive Immunology Serono Symposis Publications. New York, Raven Press, 1993, vol 97, pp 217–220.
45 Szekeres-Bartho J, Par G, Dombay G, Smart YC, Volgyi Z: The anti-abortive effect of PIBF in mice is manifested by modulating NK activity. Cell Immunol 1997;177:194–198.

Julia Szekeres-Bartho MD PhD
Professor of Microbilogy
Department of Medical Microbiology & Immunology
Medical School, Pecs University
12 Szigeti Str, H-7643 Pecs (Hungary)
Tel. +36 72 536262, Fax +36 72 536253

Markert UR (ed): Immunology of Pregnancy.
Chem Immunol Allergy. Basel, Karger, 2005, vol 89, pp 126–134

Regeneration and Tolerance Factor

A Vacuolar ATPase with Consequences

Rita F. Levine, Richards Derks, Kenneth Beaman

Clinical Immunology Laboratory, Rosalind Franklin University of Medicine and Science, North Chicago, Ill., USA

Abstract

Embryonic-maternal signaling is vital to implantation. We have identified a cellular protein that indirectly regulates secretion of IL-1β, a proinflammatory cytokine that is involved in this signaling process. Regeneration and tolerance factor is a V-ATPase protein that regulates ATP levels in a variety of cells including macrophages, which, in turn, regulates the P2X7 ligand-gated ion channel. As extracellular levels of ATP rise, the P2X7 receptor undergoes a change in permeability, which leads to the onset of apoptotic events and the release of IL-1β. IL-1β leads to local inflammation and vascularization, which is integral to establishing a successful implantation site.

Introduction

A successful pregnancy requires both a viable blastocyst that is capable of implanting in the uterus and a receptive endometrium. How a mother and an embryo participate in and contribute to these two requirements has been the subject of much inquiry and research over the years. While the regulatory role of ovarian and pituitary hormones has been well documented, recent research suggests additional regulatory factors. One such factor is embryonic-maternal signaling through the presence and activity of growth factors and cytokines [1–3]. We are particularly interested in a specific cytokine, interleukin-1β (IL-1β) because of its ability to initiate inflammation and the subsequent vascularization of the endometrium. This vascularization is necessary for implantation to proceed. Factors that participate in the production and release of IL-1β include regeneration and tolerance factor (RTF), which is a vacuolar ATPase, and the P2X7 purinoceptor. The relationship that exists between these proteins and their relevance to pregnancy is the topic of this manuscript.

IL-1 Cytokines and Pregnancy

IL-1β cytokine is present at the maternal-fetal interface in a number of mammals. In humans, mRNA for IL-1β has been found in endometrial tissue [4], and active IL-1β has been detected in endometrial macrophages, endothelial cells, and leukocytes [5]. Human preimplantation embryos also produce IL-1α and IL-1β [6, 7]. Similarly, in mice, both mRNA for IL-1α and IL-1β as well as the proteins themselves are detected in high levels in uterine tissue just prior to implantation [8]. Examination of developing embryos reveals that 4-cell embryos are the first to contain mRNA for IL-1β, and that mRNA is present up through to the blastocyst stage [1]. IL-1 type 1 receptors in mice were localized in the maternal lumenal epithelium, and during periimplantation (day 4 in mice) type 1 receptors were evident in the epithelium surrounding the blastocyst [5]. Mated mice treated with IL-1 receptor antagonist during the first 9 days of gestation failed to achieve pregnancy [9]. Other studies that examined matings of mice that lacked the IL-1 type 1 receptor resulted in relatively normal implantation and pregnancy [10] as did matings between IL-1β knockout mice [11]. This suggests that embryonic IL-1β signaling may not be imperative for implantation.

Two forms of IL-1, IL-1α and IL-1β, mediate inflammation and share the same cell surface receptors [12]. IL-1α is membrane bound and IL-1β is a soluble protein [13]. Two IL-1 receptors have been identified, along with a natural receptor antagonist [14]. When the type 1 receptor binds IL-1β, signal transduction occurs, while the type 2 receptor lacks any known function. Both IL-1α and IL-1β are synthesized as 31-kDa precursors and are secreted as 17-kDa active proteins. IL-1β must be proteolytically cleaved by caspase-1 (ICE, IL-1β-converting enzyme) to become a biologically active protein [15]. This cleavage requires the external activation of another membrane receptor, P2X7 [16], which will be discussed shortly. Unlike most secreted proteins, IL-1β lacks a hydrophobic leader sequence [17]. Therefore, it does not enter the endoplasmic reticulum and Golgi complex for processing the way that most secretory proteins do [18, 19]. For years, the exact mechanism of IL-1β secretion was unknown; however, recent research has revealed new insights into its release [20–22].

RTF and Pregnancy

Another protein that is present at the maternal-fetal interface and plays a role in implantation is RTF. We have shown that RTF participates in and regulates

IL-1β secretion [23]. RTF was originally cloned from a mouse T cell line [24]. Early treatment of mated mice with antibody to RTF prevented pregnancy [25], suggesting that RTF has a role in reproduction. In humans, the pattern of RTF expression can be used as a diagnostic indicator of a successful pregnancy. When compared to nonpregnant controls, RTF is upregulated on B cells (CD19+) from pregnant women, but not T cells (CD3+). In addition, women who experience recurrent, spontaneous abortions have NK cells (CD56+) with surface RTF [26]. RTF is present on the cell surface of a number of cell types including placental cells [27, 28], T cells, B cells, macrophages [29], and regenerating hepatocytes [30]. It is also present on B cell lymphocytic leukemia cells [31], choriocarcinoma cell lines, and ovarian cancer cell lines, such as OVCAR-3 and ES-2.

Using computer analysis, RTF is proposed to be a transmembrane protein that spans the plasma membrane 7 times, with an intracellular C-terminus and an extracellular N-terminus [24]. RTF is expressed in two forms, a 70-kDa protein that is found intracellularly and a 50-kDa protein that is present on the cell surface. It is believed that as the 70-kDa RTF comes to the surface of the cell, a 20-kDa N-terminal portion is cleaved off at a serine protease site [24].

RTF Is a V-ATPase

RTF shares 100% amino acid sequence homology with the α2 isoform of the α subunit of vacuolar H^+-adenosine triphosphatase (V-ATPase) [32]. V-ATPases are enzymes present in vacuolar organelles and in the plasmalemma of specialized cells [33]. The surface form of vacuolar ATPase is responsible for hydrolyzing extracellular adenosine triphosphate (ATP). V-ATPase is composed of two multisubunit domains. There is a transmembrane domain, which is responsible for proton translocation, and a peripheral, catalytic domain that extends into the extracellular matrix and is responsible for ATP hydrolysis [34]. The α subunit of V-ATPase is a glycoprotein that spans the membrane with 6–8 helices [35]. The α subunit may allow for proton translocation to other subunits and may be important for assembly of the V-ATPase protein [36]. This enzyme requires ATP to pump protons across intracellular membranes. This creates a pH gradient that leads to acidification within the intracellular compartments while the cytosol remains neutral [37]. V-ATPases are responsible for energizing the plasma membrane in animal cells and are as important as Na^+K^+ ATPases [37, 38]. In macrophages and neutrophils, V-ATPases maintain a neutral environment in the cytosol [39, 40]. Increasing levels of V-ATPases in the plasma membrane of neutrophils have been shown to delay apoptosis [41]. V-ATPases are also functionally expressed in a variety of human tumor cells and may have specialized roles in cell growth and metastasis [42–45].

As V-ATPase, RTF is present in an intracellular form as well as an extracellular form embedded in the plasma membrane. We demonstrated that the 50-kDa surface form is a functional ATPase by using antibody to RTF to block ATP hydrolysis. Human peripheral blood mononuclear cells (PBMC) that were incubated with anti-RTF had a 10-fold decrease in surface ATPase activity when compared to PBMCs treated with an isotype control antibody [46]. RTF's ability to hydrolyze extracellular ATP in turn regulates the P2X7 receptor. We believe that this is the method for the production and release of mature, bioactive IL-1β.

P2X7 Ion Channels

P2X7 receptors are part of a family of ion channels that bind nucleotides [47]. P2X7 receptors are present primarily on cells of hemopoietic origin, such as T cells, B cells, macrophages, and monocytes, as well as epithelial cells [48, 49]. Upon binding extracellular ATP, the plasma membrane undergoes a change in permeability, initially allowing an influx of small ions such as Ca^{2+} into the cell through selective channels. K^+ ions then exit the cell. If ATP exposure is prolonged, larger cations and hydrophobic molecules 600–900 Da enter into the cell through nonselective channels [50]. Activation of P2X7 receptors leads to activation of caspases [51], which leads to apoptosis [52, 53]. The activation of the P2X7 receptor by extracellular ATP is also connected with the release of IL-1β. Studies in mice lacking functional P2X7 receptors were unable to produce IL-1β upon stimulation with ATP [54, 55].

RTF, Apoptosis and Cellular Activation

Work in our lab has focused on how RTF regulates apoptosis. We have studied apoptosis in human PBMC, purified T cells, T cell lines (Jurkat and THP-1) and macrophage lines (J774). We measured annexin V binding to phosphatidyl-serine residues on the cell surface, DNA fragmentation, as well as caspase 3 activation, and uptake of propidium iodide as indicators of apoptosis. We found that T cells and macrophages that were treated with antibody directed against RTF underwent apoptosis at significantly higher rates than cells treated with isotype-matched control antibody [46, 56, 57]. The addition of ATP to cells treated with anti-RTF antibody resulted in increased apoptosis. When ATPase was added to cells treated with anti-RTF antibody and ATP, no apoptosis occurred. This demonstrated that RTF regulates surface ATPase activity and binding of ATP to the P2X7 receptor. By regulating the amount of extracellular ATP available to bind P2X7, RTF regulates apoptosis.

Further studies demonstrated that the amount of apoptosis that occurred was directly related to the levels of surface RTF as opposed to intracellular RTF [46]. The state of activation of the cell was also found to be highly significant with respect to RTF expression. RTF was analyzed by Western blot that had been probed with anti-RTF antibody. Resting human PBMC were examined for RTF on their cells. Normal cells express both forms of RTF; however, the 70-kDa intracellular form was far more prevalent than the 50-kDa surface form [46]. Upon cell activation, the surface form of RTF was upregulated [23]. In vitro activation of T cells and PBMC was achieved by incubating cells with anti-CD3ε and/or anti-CD28 antibody. An interesting time course display of RTF emerged. Prior to activation, PBMC display mostly 70-kDa RTF. Following activation with anti-CD3ε and anti-CD28 antibody, RTF levels were undetectable for 16–24 h. After 24–48 h RTF became measurable; however, now the predominant form was the 50-kDa surface form of the protein [23, 46].

We also examined RTF mRNA during this same time period and found that in resting cells the amount of mRNA was at the highest level seen. This high level of mRNA continued when RTF was undetectable in the cell and the amount of mRNA began to drop as the 50-kDa surface form became predominant. The consequence of this RTF shift was evident in V-ATPase activity and apoptotic activity of activated cells. Unstimulated PBMC demonstrated low levels of apoptosis when treated with anti-RTF antibody and no apoptosis was seen in cells 16–24 h after stimulation when treated with anti-RTF antibody. Higher levels of apoptosis were measured at 48 and 72 h when the 50-kDa surface form of RTF was predominant [46].

RTF and IL-1β

Our most recent work takes the next step and demonstrates the effect RTF exerts upon IL-1β secretion. We used the macrophage cell line THP-1, which expresses both RTF and P2X7 on the cell surface. THP-1 cells were incubated with lipopolysaccharide and PBMC that were first activated with phytohemagglutinin, which we found to be necessary for the production of pro-IL-1β. As shown in figure 1, when these activated THP-1 cells were treated with ATP they released IL-1β into their culture supernatants in levels dependent on the concentration of ATP. Adding anti-RTF antibody along with ATP to activated THP-1 cells resulted in significantly higher levels of IL-1β being released by these cells. Adding ATPase along with the anti-RTF antibody and ATP to activated THP-1 cells brought the levels of IL-1β back down to those of cells treated with just ATP alone.

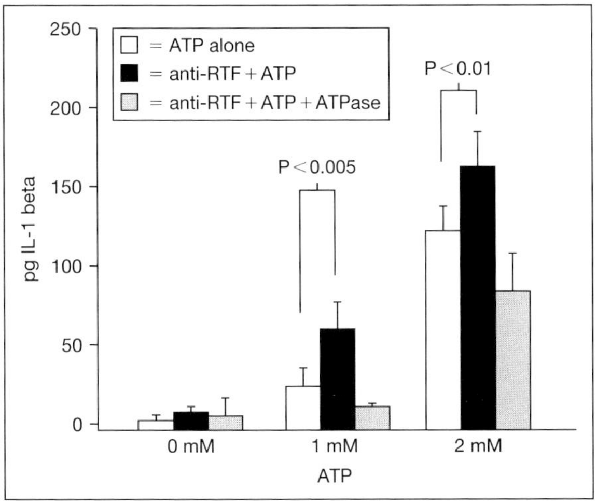

Fig. 1. RTF regulates IL-1β secretion in macrophages. IL-1β secretion of THP-1 cells incubated with varying concentrations of ATP alone, ATP + anti-RTF, or ATP + anti-RTF + ATPase is shown. Levels of IL-1β were assayed by ELISA. Bars represent standard error of the mean. Statistical significance is indicated.

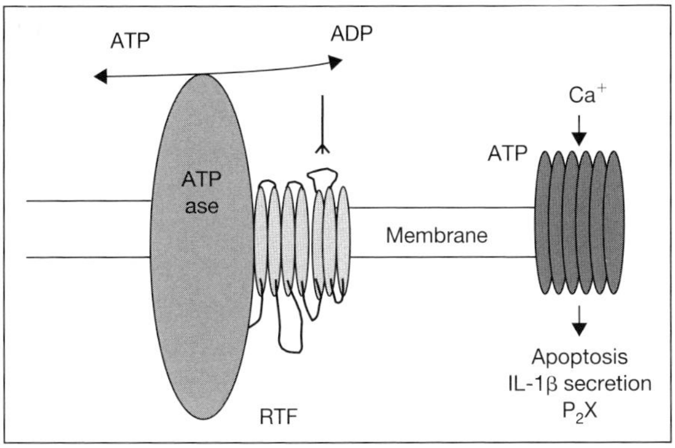

Fig. 2. Model of RTF function.

From these studies we conclude the following (please refer to fig. 2 for a schematic representation). RTF is an important membrane protein that hydrolyzes ATP. By regulating the amount of ATP available at the cell surface, RTF regulates P2X7 activation, which in turn controls apoptosis and IL-1β production and secretion. In other words, upregulation of RTF leads to decreased levels of extracellular ATP, which leads to less activation of P2X7 receptors.

This leads to less apoptosis and less IL-1β production. Downregulation of RTF leads to increased apoptosis and increased production of IL-1β. The presence of these proteins at the maternal-fetal interface indicates that RTF regulates these processes, thereby regulating implantation. These data provide a mechanism to explain the antipregnancy effect of anti-RTF antibody [58].

References

1 Takacs P, Kauma S: The expression of interleukin-1 alpha, interleukin-1 beta, and interleukin-1 receptor type I mRNA during preimplantation mouse development. J Reprod Immunol 1996; 32/1:27.

2 Sharkey A: Cytokines and implantation. Rev Reprod 1998;3:52.

3 Robertson SA, Redman CW, McCracken SA, Hunt JS, Dimitriadis E, Moffett-King A, Chamely L: Immune modulators of implantation and placental development – A workshop report. Placenta 2003;24(suppl A):S16–S20.

4 Kauma S, Matt D, Strom S, Eierman D, Turner T: Interleukin-1 beta, human leukocyte antigen HLA-DR alpha, and transforming growth factor-beta expression in endometrium, placenta and placental membranes. Am J Obstet Gynecol 1990;163:1430.

5 Simon C, Piquette G, Frances A, Polan M: Localization of interleukin-1 type receptor and interleukin-1b in human endometrium throughout the menstrual cycle. J Clin Endocrinol Metab 1993; 77:549.

6 Zolti M, Ben-Rafael Z, Meirom R, Shemesh M, Bider D, Mashiach S, Apte R: Cytokine involvement in oocytes and early embryos. Fertil Steril 1991;56:265.

7 De los Santos M, Mercader A, Frances A, Portoles E, Remohf J, Pellicer A: Immunoreactive human embryonic interleukin-1 system and endometrial factors regulating their secretion during embryonic development. Biol Reprod 1996;54:563.

8 De M, Sanford TR, Wood GW: Expression of interleukin 1, interleukin 6 and tumour necrosis factor alpha in mouse uterus during the peri-implantation period of pregnancy. J Reprod Fertil 1993; 97/1:83.

9 Simon C, Frances A, Piquette G, Danasouri I, Zurawski G, Dang W, Polan M: Embryonic implantation in mice is blocked by interleukin-1 receptor antagonist. Endocrinology 1994; 134:521.

10 Abbondanzo S, Cullinan E, McIntyre K, Labow M, Stewart C: Reproduction in mice lacking a functional type 1 IL-1 receptor. Endocrinology 1996;137:3598.

11 Zheng L, Conejo-Garcia JR, Katsaros D, Gimotty PA, Massobrio M, Regnani G, Makrigiannakis A, Gray H, Schlienger K, Liebman MN, Rubin SC, Coukos G: Intratumoral T cells, recurrence, and survival in epithelial ovarian cancer. N Engl J Med 2003;348/3:203.

12 Dower SK, Kronheim SR, Hopp TP, Cantrell M, Deeley M, Gillis S, Henney CS, Urdal DL: The cell surface receptors for interleukin-la and interleukin-lb are identical. Nature 1986; 324:266.

13 Lepe-Zuniga B, Gery I: Production of intracellular and extracellular interleukin-1 by human monocytes. Clin Immunol Immunopathol 1984;31:222.

14 Dinarello C: Interleukin-1 and interleukin-1 antagonism. Blood 1991;77:1627.

15 Dinarello C: Biologic basis of interleukin-1 in disease. Blood 1996;87:2095.

16 Ferrari D, Los M, Bauer M, Vandenabeele P, Wesselborg S, Schulze-Osthoff K: P2Z purinoreceptor ligation induces activation of caspases with distinct roles in apoptotic and necrotic alteration of cell death. FEBS Lett 1999;447:71–75.

17 March C, Mosley B, Larson A, Cerretti D, Braedt B, Price V, Gillis S, Henney C, Kronheim S, Grabstein K, Conlon P, Hopp T, Cosman D: Cloning, sequence and expression of two distinct human interleukin 1 complementary DNAs. Nature 1985;315:641.

18 Singer II, Scott S, Hall G, Limjuco G, Chin J, Schmidt J: Interleukin 1 beta is localized in the cytoplasmic ground substance but is largely absent from the Golgi apparatus and plasma membrane of stimulated human monocytes. J Exp Med 1988;167:389.

19 Rubatelli A, Sitia R: Secretion of mammalian proteins that lack a signal sequence; in Kuchler K, Rubatelli A, Holland B (eds): Usual Secretory Pathways: From Bateria to Man. Austin, Landes, 1997, p 87.
20 MacKenzie A, Wilson H, Kiss-Toth E, Dower S, North A, Surprenant A: Rapid secretion of interleukin-1b by microvesicle shedding. Immunity 2001;8:825.
21 Gudipaty L, Munetz J, Verhoef P, Dubyak G: Essential role for Ca^{2+} in regulation of IL-1beta secretion by P2X7 nucleotide receptor in monocytes, macrophages and HEK-293 cell. Am J Physiol 2003;285:C286.
22 Brough D, Feuvre RL, Wheeler R, Solovyova N, Hilfiker S, Rothwell N, Verkhratsky A: Ca^{2+} stores and Ca^{2+} entry differentially contribute to the release of IL-1 beta and IL-1 alpha from murine macrophages. J Immunol 2003;170:3029.
23 Derks R, Beaman K: Regeneration and tolerance factor modulates the effect of ATP induced IL-1b secretion in human macrophages. Hum Immunol 2004;65:676.
24 Lee C, Ghoshal K, Beaman KD: Cloning of a cDNA for a T cell produced molecule with a putative immune regulatory role. Mol Immunol 1990;27:1137.
25 Ribbing SL, Hoversland RC, Beaman KD: T cell suppressor factors play an integral role in preventing fetal rejection. J Reprod Immunol 1988;14:83.
26 Nichols TC, Kang JA, Angkachatchi V, Beer AE, Beaman KD: Expression of a membrane form of the pregnancy-associated protein TJ6 on lymphocytes. Cell Immunol 1994;155:219.
27 Lee GW, Boomer JS, Gilman-Sachs A, Chedid A, Gudelj L, Rukavina D, Beaman KD: Regeneration and tolerance factor of the human placenta induces IL-10 production. Eur J Immunol 2001;31:687.
28 Rubesa G, Beaman KD, Lucin P, Rukavina D: Expression of RTF protein in the human first trimester decidual lymphocytes. Reg Immunol 1994;6:331.
29 Mandal M, Beaman KD: Purification and characterization of a pregnancy associated protein from the feto-placental unit. Am J Reprod Immunol 1994;33:60.
30 Chedid A, Sung CC, Lepe MR, Ahmed SA, Iftikhar SA, Feller A, Beaman KD: Expression of a novel protein by regenerating hepatocytes and peripheral blood lymphocytes. Clin Diagn Lab Immunol 2001;8:1292.
31 Aslakson CJ, Lee GW, Gilman-Sachs A, Kucuk O, Beaman KD: Regeneration and tolerance factor is expressed on leukemias and may be a mechanism for leukemias to escape immune surveillance. Am J Hematol 1999;61:46.
32 Toyomura T, Oka T, Yamaguchi C, Wada Y, Futai M: Three subunit a isoforms of mouse vacuolar H^+-ATPase. J Biol Chem 2000;275:8760.
33 Gluck S: V-ATPases of the plasma membrane. J Exp Biol 1992;172:29.
34 Forgac M: Structure function and regulation of the vacuolar (H^+)-ATPases. FEBS Lett 1998; 440:258.
35 Perin M, Fried V, Stone K, Xie X, Sudhof T: Structure of the 116-kDa polypeptide of the clathrin-coated vesicle/synaptic vesicle proton pump. J Biol Chem 1991;266:3877–3881.
36 Leng X, Manolson M, Liu Q, Forgac M: Site directed mutagenesis of the 100 kDa subunit (Vphlp) of the yeast vacuolar (H^+)-ATPase. J Biol Chem 1996;271:22487.
37 Nelson N: The vacuolar H^+-ATPases. J Exp Biol 1992;172:19.
38 Wieczorek H, Brown D, Grinstein S, Ehrenfeld J, Harvey W: Energization of animal plasma membranes by proton-motive V-ATPase. Bioassays 1999;21:637.
39 Swallow C, Grinstein S, Rotstein O: A vacuolar type (H^+)-ATPase regulates cytoplasmic pH in murine macrophages. J Biol Chem 1990;265:7645.
40 Swallow C, Grinstein S, Sudsbury R, Rotstein O: Relative roles of Na^+/H^+ exchange and vacuolar-type H^+ ATPases in regulating cytoplasmic pH and function in murine peritoneal macrophages. J Cell Physiol 1993;157:453.
41 Gottlieb R, Giesing H, Zhu J, Engler R, Babior B: Cell acidification in apoptosis granulocyte colony-stimulating factor delays programmed cell death in neutrophils by up-regulating the vacuolar H^+-ATPase. Proc Natl Acad Sci USA 1995;92:5965.
42 Martinez-Zaguilan R, Martinez G, Gomez A, Hendrix M, Gillies R: Distinct regulation of pH and Ca^{2+} in human melanoma cells with different metastatic potential. J Cell Physiol 1998; 176:196.

43 Martinez-Zaguilan R, Raghunand N, Lynch RM, Bellamy W, Martinez GM, Rojas B, Smith D, Dalton WS, Gillies RJ: pH and drug resistance. I. Functional expression of plasmalemmal V-type H^+-ATPase in drug-resistant human breast carcinoma cell lines. Biochem Pharmacol 1999;57:1037.
44 Sennoune S, Luo D, Martinez-Zaguilan R: Plasmalemmal vacuolar-type H^+-ATPase in cancer biology. Cell Biochem Biophys 2004;40:185.
45 Sennoune S, Bakunts K, Martinez G, Chua-Tuan J, Kebir Y, Attaya M, Martinez-Zaguilan R: Vacuolar H^+-ATPase in human breast cancer cells with distinct metastatic potential: Distribution and functional activity. Am J Physiol 2004;286:C1443–C1452.
46 Derks R, Beaman KD: Regeneration and tolerance factor (RTF) prevents bystander T cell death associated with HIV infection. Clin Diagn Lab Immunol 2004;11:835–840.
47 North A: Molecular physiology of P2X receptors. Physiol Rev 2002;82:1013.
48 Collo G, Neidhart S, Kawashima E, Kosco-Vilbois R, North A, Buell G: Tissue distribution of the P2X7 receptor. Neuropharmacology 1997;36:1277.
49 DiVirgilio F, Chiozzi P, Ferrari D, Falzoni S, Sanz J, Morelli Z, Torboli M, Bolognesi F, Baricordi R: Nucleotide receptors: An emerging family of regulatory molecules in blood cells. Blood 2001; 97:587.
50 DiVirgilio F: The P2Z purinoceptor: An intriguing role in immunity, inflammation and cell death. Immunol Today 1995;16:524.
51 Martin SJ, Green DR: Protease activation during apoptosis: Death by a thousand cuts? Cell 1995; 82:349.
52 Ferrari D, Chiozzi P, Falzoni S, Susino MD, Melchiorri L, Baricordi OR, Virgilio FD: Extracellular ATP triggers IL-1 beta release by activating the purinergic P2Z receptor of human macrophages. J Immunol 1997;159:1451–1458.
53 Schulze-Lohoff E, Hugo C, Rost S, Arnold S, Gruber A, Brune B, Sterzel RB: Extracellular ATP causes apoptosis and necrosis of cultured mesangial cells via P2Z/P2X_7 receptors. Am J Physiol 1998;275:F962.
54 Labasi J, Petrushova N, Donovan C, McCurdy S, Lira P, Payette M, Brissette W, Wicks J, Audoly L, Gabel C: Absence of the P2X7 receptor alters leukocyte function and attenuates and inflammatory response. J Immunol 2002;168:6436.
55 Solle M, Labasi J, Perregauz G, Stam E, Petrushova N, Koller B, Griffiths R, Gabel C: Altered cytokine production in mice lacking P2X7 receptors. J Biol Chem 2001;276:126.
56 Boomer JS, Lee GW, Givens TS, Gilman-Sachs A, Beaman KD: Regeneration and tolerance factors' potential role in T cell activation and apoptosis. Hum Immunol 2000;61:959.
57 Boomer JS, Derks RA, Lee GW, DuChateau BK, Gilman-Sachs A, Beaman KD: Regeneration and tolerance factor (RTF) is expressed during T lymphocyte activation and plays a role in apoptosis. Hum Immunol 2001;62:577.
58 Beaman KD, Hoversland RC: Induction of abortion in mice with a monoclonal antibody specific for suppressor T-lymphocyte molecules. J Reprod Immunol 1988;14:83.

Kenneth Beaman,
Clinical Immunology Laboratory, Rosalind Franklin University of Medicine and Science
3333 Green Bay Road,
North Chicago, IL 60064 (USA)
Tel. +1 847 578 8832, Fax +1 847 775 6506
E-Mail Kenneth.Beaman@rosalindfranklin.edu

Market UR (ed): Immunology of Pregnancy.
Chem Immunol Allergy. Basel, Karger, 2005, vol 89, pp 135–148

Nerve Growth Factor in Reproductive Biology: Link between the Immune, Endocrine and Nervous System?

Mareike Tometten, Sandra Blois, Petra C. Arck

Charité, University Medicine Berlin, Berlin, Germany

Abstract

Successful pregnancy outcome requires balanced networking of the immune and endocrine system. In addition, numerous sophisticated adaptive mechanisms promote invasion of fetal tissue and facilitate tolerance. This highly sensitive and vulnerable environment may be challenged from either the maternal or the fetal site. In this overview we collect evidence of a functional role of neurotrophins, predominately nerve growth factor (NGF), in pregnancy maintenance. We demonstrate several pathways through which NGF may be involved in maintaining pregnancy and/or – if exaggerated – inducing pregnancy failure. Due to the pleiotropism of NGF, we hypothesize that NGF is mandatory for the success of pregnancy, e.g. via inhibition of paternal MHC II molecule expression on trophoblast cells. This is supported by published evidence on progesterone, the hormone of pregnancy, which maintains local levels of NGF. On the other hand, if levels of NGF are upregulated in response to environmental challenges, e.g. stress, this may result in a threat to pregnancy maintenance due to a skew towards proinflammatory cytokines and increased apoptotic cell death. Hence, we strongly suggest that NGF constitutes a functional link between the nervous, endocrine and immune system translating environmental or endocrine signals during pregnancy into an immunological answer.

Introduction

Reproductive success constitutes a major feat and need for species conservation. In mammalian pregnancies, a nutritious environment for growth and development of the fetus is compulsory, but maternal immune responses against fetal alloantigens ought to be suppressed to avoid rejection. For tolerance of the allograft, adaptation of the uterine environment is required. Thus, successful pregnancy implies exceeding coordination and adjustment to divers complex biological processes, including endocrine, vascular, metabolic and immune functions.

In the present overview, we highlight the role of neurotrophins (NTs), a chameleonic family of proteins, as a potent mediator within the coordinative network of successful and/or adverse pregnancy outcome. Nerve growth factor (NGF) was the first identified member of the NTs, and in the past decades, the existence of additional members of this family has emerged, including the brain-derived neurotrophic factor (BDNF), neurotrophin-3 (NT-3) and neurotrophin-4/5 (NT-4/5) [1]. NTs represent a family of polypeptide growth factors that have similarities in structure, receptor utility as well as physiological activities, and are essential for the development of the vertebrate nervous system. They regulate survival, death or differentiation of neurons in embryonic and postnatal stages as well as neuronal maintenance later in life. For signal transduction all members of NTs use two different types of cell surface receptors: the high-affinity tropomyosin-related tyrosine kinase (trk) receptors and the low-affinity NT receptor p75NTR [2, 3].

Originally, the role of NTs was considered to be limited to the nervous system. However, a wealth of recent data indicates that NTs exert actions in a wide variety of tissues outside the nervous system including the reproductive organs [4]. NGF is now considered to maintain balanced interactions between the nervous, immune and endocrine systems, since – beside the nervous system – NGF receptor expression and responsiveness to NGF are found in a variety of immune and endocrine cells [5].

In reproductive systems, NTs are considered as critical components due to their role in the acquisition of ovarian reproductive competence. NGF promotes ovarian development by maintaining ovarian innervation and by predifferative and proliferative effects on ovarian cells. It also participates in processes involved in follicular rupture at the time of first ovulation [reviewed in 6]. In male reproductive systems, NTs and their receptors are considered to play complex autocrine or paracrine roles in both testicular development and spermatogenesis [7, 8].

Decidualization and NGF

Decidualization implies a highly specialized, endocrinologically controlled process which begins in the luteal phase of every menstrual cycle in primates. Typically, the presence and invasion of immunocompetent cells accompany and regulate this transformation. Via a distinct cytokine profile, these cells may contribute to the specialized decidual microenvironment, providing essential tolerance mechanisms for the protection of the fetal graft. We refrain from reviewing details on distinct microenvironmental cell populations, cell migration, antigen presentation or Th1/Th2 profiles in our contribution and refer to the relevant chapters in this book. Predominance of Th2 cytokines seems to be required to ensure fetal tolerance. Emerging evidence indicates that also neural factors are involved in the regulation of the Th1/Th2 balance. Being in a key position, the potent functions of NGF and other NTs in the responsiveness of immunocompetent cells are known by now [reviewed in 5, 9, 10], which strongly suggests that NTs could also act on decidual immune cells. This is based on observations indicating that lymphocytes both synthesize and release NTs and express NT receptors, which proposes autocrine and/or paracrine actions. Murine CD4+ and CD8+ T cell clones express NGF and functional trkA receptor, which is increasingly inducible by antigenic stimulation. Further, both human Th1 and Th2 cells have been demonstrated to express NGF and trkA. Interestingly, one study demonstrated a selective expression for NGF, trkA and trkC receptor in Th2 cells [11]. NT-3, which has the highest affinity for trkC, was found to enhance IL-4 production by stimulated Th2 cells suggesting that NT-3 induced a Th2 skew in these cells. In B lymphocytes, trkA and p75NTR as well as NGF expression has been reported mediating proliferation and survival of B cells with subsequent stimulation of immunoglobulin production. Mast cells synthesize, store and – during degranulation (=activation) – release biologically active NGF, e.g. in allergic responses. NGF enhances local mast cell numbers and has chemotactic effects on the respective cells. Since mast cells have been found in human and murine decidua [12, 13] and may further be innervated by peripheral neurons, NGF might participate in the regulation of cross talk between nerves and mast cells also in the context of decidualization [for a review, see 9].

Further, we know from experiments on human palatine tonsils and lymph nodes that trkA and p75NTR, but not NGF are present on dendritic cells (DCs) suggesting that lymphocyte-derived NGF could act as mediator of the cell-cell communication between lymphocytes and DCs [14]. A wealth of data now points towards the importance of identifying mediators which regulate decidual DCs, e.g. lineage or maturation [15]. Hence, future research is urgently required to identify the influence of NTs on DCs.

Monocytes express trkA and the expression increases after activation, whereas it is downregulated during differentiation towards macrophages. However, macrophages express NGF and both trkA and p75NTR, and in vitro studies revealed stimulation of TNF-α production by NGF pointing towards an activating function on macrophages during inflammatory responses [16]. NGF stimulates the secretion of other cytokines, i.e. IL-1 and IL-6. Cytokines in turn, such as TNF-α, IL-1β, IL-6, IFN-γ and transforming growth factor-β (TGF-β), are strong inducers of NGF production [5]. The level of NGF rises substantially in inflamed tissue secondary to an initial rise in the level of IL-1β.

Recent data indicate that interactional processes between NGF and immune cells could be primarily mediated by activation of endothelial cells. NGF was demonstrated to induce expression of ICAM-1 on endothelial cells, and accumulation of neutrophilic leukocytes attracted by NGF was inhibited by treatment with specific antibodies against NGF in the skin [17].

Taken together, dependent on the type of inflammation and its stage, NGF is promiscuous, possibly similar to IL-6, since it may act as an inducer of a pro- or anti-inflammatory response. However, clear evidence exists that NGF constitutes an autocrine and/or paracrine factor in the development and regulation of immune responses and is part of an integrated neuroimmune adaptive response.

The association between pregnancy-induced immune responses and NTs is based on the presence of NGF and its functional receptor trkA in decidual cells [18, 19]. In a disturbed pregnancy, e.g. upon stress exposure, both NGF- and trkA-expressing decidual cells are upregulated. Increased levels of NGF contribute to the deleterious shift of cytokines from protective Th2 (IL-4, IL-10) to inflammatory Th1 (TNF-α, IFN-γ and IL-12) which can be abrogated by the treatment of mice with an adequate dose of neutralizing NGF antibodies. Moreover, in disturbed pregnancies NGF mRNA levels increase, which is abolished by pretreatment with neutralizing antibodies against adhesion molecules ICAM-1/LFA-1 [Tometten et al., unpubl. data]. The presence of NGF and its functional receptor in uterine tissue of normally progressing and adverse pregnancy points towards a regulatory role, expanding NGF functions also in pregnancy-related physiologies and pathophysiologies. As a linking molecule between nervous, endocrine and immune system, NGF may mediate cross talk between the distinctive systems in reproductive maintenance. Based on the currently available literature we suggest that moderate levels of NGF contribute to a balanced Th2 cytokine profile while high NGF expression, as seen in response to stress, aggravates the increase of abortogenic, inflammatory cytokines. Additionally, the predominance of Th1 cytokines then leads to increased decidual NGF and trkA expression. Observations of functional effects between NGF and ICAM-1/-LFA-1 point towards a proximate NT-mediated activation of endothelial cells with subsequent recruitment of Th1 cells into the decidua.

Neurotrophins and Apoptosis at the Fetomaternal Interface

Apoptosis is an important mechanism for invasion of the developing embryo during implantation and remodeling of the maternal decidual tissue. By limiting lymphocyte proliferation following activation, programmed cell death has been proposed as one further mechanism to maintain the immunologically privileged situation at the fetomaternal interface [20, 21]. After cells have undergone programmed cell death, the apoptotic cell bodies are phagocytosed by macrophages without inducing an inflammatory response [22]. Apoptosis occurring in human villous trophoblast is thought to participate in the regulation of placental growth and function being a normal physiological process throughout gestation [23, 24].

Regulation of apoptosis is a complex process involving a family of related proteins that can exert promotive or inhibitory functions [for reviews, see 25, 26]. A prototypical member of cell death surface receptors is Fas (CD95) which mediates apoptosis through binding to its ligand FasL [20, 21, 27]. Fas-FasL interactions function to protect immune-privileged organs, and expression of FasL by placental cells may contribute to the immune-privileged status of the conceptus by protecting itself against maternal leukocytic influx [20, 26]. Also, TNF-α and IFN-γ, expressed in placental tissue, are involved in apoptotic mechanisms: cytotrophoblasts undergo apoptosis after TNF-α exposure, which is enhanced by IFN-γ [28–30].

Further ligand-receptor systems belonging to the apoptosis-mediating family are NTs and low-affinity NT receptor p75NTR. NGF has been detected and isolated from murine and human placental tissue [31]. Moreover, p75NTR has been demonstrated to be coexpressed in human placental tissue suggesting functional roles in this organ compartment [32]. The p75NTR is a member of the TNF receptor/Fas/CD40 superfamily and binds all the NTs with low affinity. The functional role of p75NTR still remains unclear: it is assumed to function as a coreceptor for the high-affinity receptors and as a mediator of proapoptotic programmes induced by NGF, depending on the physiological or developmental stage of the cells. Further, in Schwann cells and melanoma cells, p75NTR has been shown to mediate cell migration and cell invasiveness [33, 34].

Effects of NGF were investigated on trophoblastic giant cell transformation of the ectoplacental cone cells in pregnant mouse uteri showing that NGF strongly accelerated this process [18]. However, little is known on whether NGF/p75NTR exert any effects on apoptosis in the placenta. Macrophages, which are an important source for NGF synthesis, are immensely involved in the processes of programmed cell death, and p75NTR is expressed on trophoblast cells. Therefore, another possible function of NGF may be the regulatory function of physiologically occurring apoptosis. Here again, a certain level of NGF at the fetomaternal interface would be essential for progressing pregnancy.

Fetal Antigenic Immaturity

Allograft rejection is mediated by genes of the major histocompatibility complex (MHC) which include the human leukocyte antigen (HLA) genes. Though maternal-fetal HLA incompatibility is not deleterious during pregnancy, the survival of the fetal allograft in mammalian pregnancy remains a paradox. In brief (since this topic has been addressed more extensively in other chapters of this book), adaptive mechanisms concerning the expression of MHC molecules in fetal tissue include the lack of classical MHC antigens on placental cells. Instead, fetal extravillous cytotrophoblast cells, which directly contact and invade maternal uterine tissue, express an unusual combination of one classical and two nonclassical MHC I molecules, HLA-G, HLA-E and HLA-C [35–37]. Expression of HLA-G protein occurs exclusively in cells at the fetal-maternal interface. Existence of at least five isoforms suggests that there may be multiple functions of HLA-G, including antigen presentation, immunomodulation of maternal T cell populations as well as permission of fetal allograft tolerance [38, 39]. The absence of MHC II molecules on trophoblast layers appears to be an important feature for fetal survival. IFN-γ is one of the most potent inducers of MHC II antigens, which may also be applicable for trophoblastic tissue. Imbalances of the local cytokine profile with increased IFN-γ production may effect placental MHC II expression resulting in the initiation of fetal rejection [40]. Interestingly, in isolated microglia cells, MHC class II inducibility by IFN-γ is enhanced by neutralization of NTs, while the presence of NGF, BDNF or NT-3 inhibits this process [41].

Accordingly, in kinetic studies with treatment of stressed pregnant mice with neutralizing antibodies against NGF, it was observed that a moderate antibody dose had a pregnancy protective effect by lowering the abortion rate. However, animals treated with a high antibody dose presented an increased abortion rate [Tometten et al., unpubl. data]. Based on the insights of Neumann et al. [41], it could be hypothesized that depriving the microenvironment at the fetomaternal interface beyond a certain level of NGF might result in an induction of deleterious MHC II expression on trophoblast cells, further indicating that balanced NGF levels are essential for pregnancy maintenance.

Interactions between Neurotrophins and Progesterone

For successful implantation and maintenance of pregnancy, the steroidal hormone progesterone is indispensable. Adequate progesterone production by the corpus luteum, the source of progesterone, is critical for the maintenance of pregnancy until the placenta undertakes this function at 7–9 weeks of human gestation. Inadequate progesterone levels result in pregnancy loss in humans and rodents [42, 43]. Progesterone is able to lower immune responses and to displace the Th1/Th2 balance towards Th2 [44, 45]. By suppressing progesterone levels, psychoemotional stress is considered to inhibit female reproduction. Substitution of progesterone in stressed animals abrogates the abortogenic stress effects by influencing the cytokine profile towards pregnancy-protective Th2 [43, 46]. Many of the progesterone effects are mediated by progesterone-induced blocking factor. Immunological functions of progesterone-induced blocking factor include inhibition of NK cell activity and action on the cytokine balance exerting antiabortive effects.

Interactions between reproductive hormones and both NTs and their receptors in the central and peripheral nervous system are well documented [47–50]. Physiological changes in the levels of gonadal steroids affect central trkA levels and progesterone treatment upregulates NGF in rodent uterus [51, 52]. Ovariectomized mice exhibit a decreased uterine NGF protein content, while estrogen and/or progesterone treatment of the respective animals restore NGF protein levels. Keeping these effects of progesterone on NGF expression in mind, it may be assumed that progesterone regulates local NGF content in pregnant uterine tissue. This hormone-NT interplay would hence extend progesterone-protective functions in pregnancy by providing the required and balanced NGF concentration at the fetomaternal interface.

Indoleamine 2,3-Dioxygenase Expression and NGF

Additionally to immunosuppressive mechanisms at the fetomaternal interface protecting the conceptus, tryptophan catabolism has been proposed as one potential component. Indoleamine 2,3-dioxygenase (IDO) is an enzymatic protein that catabolizes tryptophan. Inhibition of IDO by application of 1-methyl-tryptophan to pregnant mice results in extensive inflammation, hemorrhagic necrosis and T cell infiltrate at the fetomaternal interface. Strikingly, transgenically altered DCs with high IDO expression lower the tryptophan concentration and suppress allogeneic T cell responses [53], possibly by depriving T cells of tryptophan [54]. IDO is synthesized and secreted by human trophoblast cells and, hence, may be required for pregnancy maintenance. Due to the IDO expression on trophoblasts, it has been suggested that the fetus protects itself by suppressing rejection by the maternal T cells. However, it has recently been revealed that mice with defective IDO genes have successful pregnancies, indicating that IDO activity is not the sole mechanism to protect the allogeneic fetus from rejection. Other mechanisms, perhaps redundant in normal mice, seem to compensate for the loss of IDO activity during gestation [55].

Besides its implication in T cell response, tryptophan has been shown to stimulate NGF production in cultured mouse astroglial cells in a dose-dependent manner [56]. No data are available about tryptophan-metabolic pathways of NGF production in immune cells. However, high tryptophan levels – due to low IDO activity in threatened pregnancies – could result in an increased local NGF production; we hypothesize that this contributes to a deleterious pregnancy course.

Adverse Pregnancy Outcome: Stress and Pregnancy Loss

Beside 'classical' causes of pregnancy loss – genetic, endocrinological, anatomic, microbiological and allo-/autoimmune causes – social-environmental influences such as stress have been linked to spontaneous abortion as an adverse reproductive outcome [57]. Increased stress perception correlates with rejection of chromosomally normal embryos, and improved stress coping by psychotherapeutic intervention results in uncomplicated pregnancy outcome. Stress-related hormones, which are partially also pregnancy related, interact with peripheral and local immune cells resulting in changes of cytokine production. By disturbing the required balanced interaction of nervous, endocrine and immune system, the effects on pregnancy induced by stress constitute considerable mechanisms in pregnancy failure [58].

In this context, the well-established concept of neurogenic inflammation ought to be mentioned. By definition, local inflammatory reactions in response to infection, toxins or trauma involve nerves which contain inflammatory neuropeptides, also referred to as neurogenic inflammation. Further, psychological or physical stress can cause neurogenic inflammatory responses by release of neuropeptides from sensory nerves and consecutive activation of mast cells and/or other immune cells. The most potent agent is neurotransmitter substance P (SP) which mediates extravasation from postcapillary venules, increases blood flow due to dilatation of arterioles and acts chemotactically on polymorphonuclear leukocytes [59]. Functional SP receptors are expressed on various immune cells including lymphocytes, macrophages, neutrophils and mast cells [60]. Effects on divers immune responses such as T cell proliferation, immunoglobulin synthesis, lymphocyte traffic, macrophage activation and mast cell degranulation as well as stimulation of cytokine production, e.g. IL-6, TNF-α and IFN-γ, are part of its functions.

Attempting to further elucidate the precise underlying mechanisms by which stress affects pregnancy, it is now well established that stress exposure during the peri-implantation period results in a decrease of pregnancy-protective Th2 cytokines and an increase of abortogenic Th1 cytokines, e.g. IL-12, TNF-α and IFN-γ [61, 62]. In humans, high stress scores in women with abortion correlate with increased numbers of local mast cells, CD8+ T cells and TNF-α-expressing cells. Further, SP is involved in the pathway of stress-induced pregnancy failure. The abortogenic Th1 cytokine profile observed in stressed pregnancies is mediated by SP-dependent pathways. Peri-implantation stress exposure of pregnant mice results in SP-mediated activation of uterine T cells, mast cells and macrophages, an increase of local TNF-α levels and a decrease of protective TGF-β.

Interactional functions between NGF and both stress and SP have been intensively studied and revealed that NGF participates in specific neuroendocrine/endocrine functions [63]. Using different stressors, several studies in humans and rodents demonstrated an increase of NGF due to stressful events, e.g. the first parachute jump, exposure to aggressive behavior or the chronic stress of caregivers. NGF is considered as an alerting signal for priming the immune system by the brain towards noxious inputs. The inflammatory milieu is characterized by high local SP and NGF levels [64, 65]. SP has been shown to directly induce NGF mRNA expression and secretion of bioactive NGF in distinct human and murine cells [66]. In turn, in vivo and in vitro studies revealed NGF as activator of SP synthesis and release, proposing a regulatory function for NGF during inflammatory processes [67]. Due to these bidirectional interactions, an interdependency between NGF and SP has been assumed pointing to a functional link between NGF and neuropeptides [68]. Recently, we could prove the hypothesis of interactional relationships between abortion induced by stress, SP and NGF. Examining decidual tissue of stressed mice, both NGF and functional trkA-expressing cells and mRNA levels are increased, which was also observed in SP-injected mice, supporting the above-mentioned insights [19]. The increase of decidual NGF caused by exposure to a stressor seems to be mediated by SP. Further, increased NGF levels after stress exposure contribute to the deleterious shift of cytokines from protective Th2 (IL-4, IL-10) to inflammatory Th1 (TNF-α, IFN-γ and IL-12). As mentioned earlier, these stress effects can be abrogated by treatment of stressed animals with an adequate dose of neutralizing NGF antibodies [Tometten et al., unpubl. data]. Taken together, these studies provide strong evidence for an additional link in the neuroimmunological pathogenesis of abortion induced by stress.

Concluding Remarks

Successful pregnancy outcome requires a balanced interplay between various systems, e.g. the immune, nervous and endocrine system. NGF may be involved in maintaining pregnancy and/or – if exaggerated – inducing pregnancy failure (fig. 1a). Due to the pleiotropism of NGF, we hypothesize that a

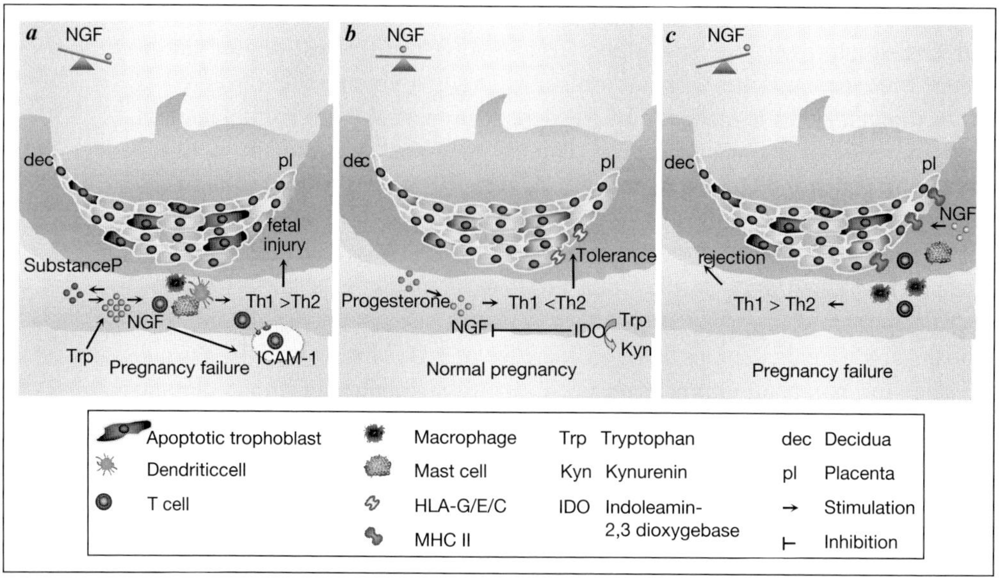

Fig. 1. Hypothetical scenario of the role of NGF in reproduction: NGF-dependent pathways. ***a*** High levels of NGF at the fetomaternal interface due to e.g. stress or high tryptophan/low IDO activity induce neurogenic inflammation, characterized by an increase of substance P, recruitment of immune cells and bias towards a Th1 cytokine profile, which results in fetal injury and rejection. ***b*** Adequate levels of NGF, possibly regulated by progesterone, contribute to the tolerogenic Th2 cytokine profile. ***c*** Deprivation of local NGF results in increased expression of abortogenic MHC II molecules on the trophoblast, hence maternal immune cells recognize and reject the fetus.

well-balanced, progesterone-mediated level of NGF is required for successful pregnancy outcome (fig. 1b). Due to its functional role, insufficient levels of NGF may provoke fetal rejection by a lack of MHC II downregulation (fig. 1c). Future work on NGF and other NTs and their respective receptors in pregnancy is urgently needed and we hope that this overview will foster recognition of NTs in basic science and clinical research in reproductive biology.

Acknowledgment

Several authors of this manuscript are members of an European Network of Excellence, entitled "EMBIC" (Embryo Implantation Control), supported by the European Union (contract no. 512040).

References

1 Levi-Montalcini R, Angeletti PU: Nerve growth factor. Physiol Rev 1968;48:534–569.

2 Lewin GR, Barde YA: Physiology of the neurotrophins. Annu Rev Neurosci 1996;19:289–317.

3 Friedman WJ, Greene LA: Neurotrophin signaling via Trks and p75. Exp Cell Res 1999; 253:131–142.

4 Tessarollo L: Pleiotropic functions of neurotrophins in development. Cytokine Growth Factor Rev 1998;9:125–137.

5 Levi-Montalcini R, Skaper SD, Dal Toso R, Petrelli L, Leon A: Nerve growth factor: From neurotrophin to neurokine. Trends Neurosci 1996;19:514–520.

6 Dissen GA, Romero C, Paredes A, Ojeda SR: Neurotrophic control of ovarian development. Microsc Res Tech 2002;59:509–515.

7 Russo MA, Giustizieri ML, Favale A, Fantini MC, Campagnolo L, Konda D, Germano F, Farini D, Manna C, Siracusa G: Spatiotemporal patterns of expression of neurotrophins and neurotrophin receptors in mice suggest functional roles in testicular and epididymal morphogenesis. Biol Reprod 1999;61:1123–1132.

8 Cupp AS, Tessarollo L, Skinner MK: Testis developmental phenotypes in neurotropin receptor trkA and trkC null mutations: Role in formation of seminiferous cords and germ cell survival. Biol Reprod 2002;66:1838–1845.

9 Aloe L, Simone MD, Properzi F: Nerve growth factor: A neurotrophin with activity on cells of the immune system. Microsc Res Tech 1999;45:285–291.

10 Bonini S, Rasi G, Bracci-Laudiero ML, Procoli A, Aloe L: Nerve growth factor: Neurotrophin or cytokine? Int Arch Allergy Immunol 2003;131:80–84.

11 Sekimoto M, Tsuji T, Matsuzaki J, Chamoto K, Koda T, Nemoto K, Degawa M, Nishimura S, Nishimura T: Functional expression of the TrkC gene, encoding a high affinity receptor for NT-3, in antigen-specific T helper type 2 (Th2) cells. Immunol Lett 2003;88:221–226.

12 Markert UR, Arck PC, McBey BA, Manuel J, Croy BA, Marshall JS, Chaouat G, Clark DA: Stress triggered abortions are associated with alterations of granulated cells into the decidua. Am J Reprod Immunol 1997;37:94–100.

13 Marx L, Arck P, Kieslich C, Mitterlechner S, Kapp M, Dietl J: Decidual mast cells might be involved in the onset of human first-trimester abortion. Am J Reprod Immunol 1999;41:34–40.

14 Garcia-Suarez O, Hannestad J, Esteban I, Martinez del Valle M, Naves FJ, Vega JA: Neurotrophin receptor-like protein immunoreactivity in human lymph nodes. Anat Rec 1997;249:226–232.

15 Blois SM, Alba Soto CD, Tometten M, Klapp BF, Margni RA, Arck PC: Lineage, maturity, and phenotype of uterine murine dendritic cells throughout gestation indicate a protective role in maintaining pregnancy. Biol Reprod 2004;70:1018–1023.

16 Barouch R, Kazimirsky G, Appel E, Brodie C: Nerve growth factor regulates TNF-alpha production in mouse macrophages via MAP kinase activation. J Leukoc Biol 2001;69:1019–1026.

17 Foster PA, Costa SK, Poston R, Hoult JR, Brain SD: Endothelial cells play an essential role in the thermal hyperalgesia induced by nerve growth factor. FASEB J 2003;17:1703–1705.

18 Kanai-Azuma M, Kanai Y, Matsuda H, Kurohmaru M, Tachi C, Yazaki K, Hayashi Y: Nerve growth factor promotes giant-cell transformation of mouse trophoblast cells in vitro. Biochem Biophys Res Commun 1997;231:309–315.

19 Tometten M, Klapp BF, Joachim R, Fest S, Zenclussen AC, Peters EM, Hertwig K, Arck PC: Nerve growth factor and its functional receptor TrkA are up-regulated in murine decidual tissue of stress-triggered and substance P-mediated abortion. Am J Reprod Immunol 2004;51:86–93.

20 Griffith TS, Ferguson TA: The role of FasL-induced apoptosis in immune privilege. Immunol Today 1997;18:240–244.

21 Lynch DH, Ramsdell F, Alderson MR: Fas and FasL in the homeostatic regulation of immune responses. Immunol Today 1995;16:569–574.

22 Mor G, Abrahams VM: Potential role of macrophages as immunoregulators of pregnancy. Reprod Biol Endocrinol 2003;1:119.

23 Hammer A, Blaschitz A, Daxbock C, Walcher W, Dohr G: Fas and Fas-ligand are expressed in the uteroplacental unit of first-trimester pregnancy. Am J Reprod Immunol 1999;41:41–51.

24 Huppertz B, Frank HG, Reister F, Kingdom J, Korr H, Kaufmann P: Apoptosis cascade progresses during turnover of human trophoblast: Analysis of villous cytotrophoblast and syncytial fragments in vitro. Lab Invest 1999;79:1687–1702.
25 Jerzak M, Bischof P: Apoptosis in the first trimester human placenta: The role in maintaining immune privilege at the maternal-foetal interface and in the trophoblast remodelling. Eur J Obstet Gynecol Reprod Biol 2002;100:138–142.
26 Levy R, Nelson DM: To be, or not to be, that is the question. Apoptosis in human trophoblast. Placenta 2000;21:1–13.
27 Nagata S: Fas and Fas ligand: A death factor and its receptor. Adv Immunol 1994;57:129–144.
28 Chen HL, Yang YP, Hu XL, Yelavarthi KK, Fishback JL, Hunt JS: Tumor necrosis factor alpha mRNA and protein are present in human placental and uterine cells at early and late stages of gestation. Am J Pathol 1991;139:327–335.
29 Bulmer JN, Morrison L, Johnson PM, Meager A: Immunohistochemical localization of interferons in human placental tissues in normal, ectopic, and molar pregnancy. Am J Reprod Immunol 1990;22:109–116.
30 Garcia-Lloret MI, Yui J, Winkler-Lowen B, Guilbert LJ: Epidermal growth factor inhibits cytokine-induced apoptosis of primary human trophoblasts. J Cell Physiol 1996;167:324–332.
31 Goldstein LD, Reynolds CP, Perez-Polo JR: Isolation of human nerve growth factor from placental tissue. Neurochem Res 1978;3:175–183.
32 MacGrogan D, Saint-Andre JP, Dicou E: Expression of nerve growth factor and nerve growth factor receptor genes in human tissues and in prostatic adenocarcinoma cell lines. J Neurochem 1992;59:1381–1391.
33 Anton ES, Weskamp G, Reichardt LF, Matthew WD: Nerve growth factor and its low-affinity receptor promote Schwann cell migration. Proc Natl Acad Sci USA 1994;91:2795–2799.
34 Herrmann JL, Menter DG, Hamada J, Marchetti D, Nakajima M, Nicolson GL: Mediation of NGF-stimulated extracellular matrix invasion by the human melanoma low-affinity p75 neurotrophin receptor: Melanoma p75 functions independently of trkA. Mol Biol Cell 1993; 4:1205–1216.
35 Le Bouteiller P: HLA class I chromosomal region, genes, and products: Facts and questions. Crit Rev Immunol 1994;14:89–129.
36 King A, Allan DS, Bowen M, Powis SJ, Joseph S, Verma S, Hiby SE, McMichael AJ Loke YW, Braud VM: HLA-E is expressed on trophoblast and interacts with CD94/NKG2 receptors on decidual NK cells. Eur J Immunol 2000;30:1623–1631.
37 King A, Burrows TD, Hiby SE, Bowen JM, Joseph S, Verma S, Lim PB, Gardner L, Le Bouteiller P, Ziegler A, Uchanska-Ziegler B, Loke YW: Surface expression of HLA-C antigen by human extravillous trophoblast. Placenta 2000;21:376–387.
38 Le Gal FA, Riteau B, Sedlik C, Khalil-Daher I, Menier C, Dausset J, Guillet JG, Carosella ED, Rouas-Freiss N: HLA-G-mediated inhibition of antigen-specific cytotoxic T lymphocytes. Int Immunol 1999;11:1351–1356.
39 Bainbridge DR, Ellis SA, Sargent IL: HLA-G suppresses proliferation of CD4(+) T-lymphocytes. J Reprod Immunol 2000;48:17–26.
40 Vassiliadis S, Tsoukatos D, Athanassakis I: Interferon-induced class II expression at the spongiotrophoblastic zone of the murine placenta is linked to fetal rejection and developmental abnormalities. Acta Physiol Scand 1994;151:485–495.
41 Neumann H, Misgeld T, Matsumuro K, Wekerle H: Neurotrophins inhibit major histocompatibility class II inducibility of microglia: Involvement of the p75 neurotrophin receptor. Proc Natl Acad Sci USA 1998;95:5779–5784.
42 Deanesly R: Termination of early pregnancy in rats after ovariectomy is due to immediate collapse of the progesterone-dependent decidua. J Reprod Fertil 1973;35:183–186.
43 Joachim R, Zenclussen AC, Polgar B, Douglas AJ, Fest S, Knackstedt M, Klapp BF, Arck PC: The progesterone derivative dydrogesterone abrogates murine stress-triggered abortion by inducing a Th2 biased local immune response. Steroids 2003;68:931–940.
44 Siiteri PK, Febres F, Clemens LE, Chang RJ, Gondos B, Stites D: Progesterone and maintenance of pregnancy: Is progesterone nature's immunosuppressant? Ann NY Acad Sci 977;286:384–397.

45 Piccinni MP, Giudizi MG, Biagiotti R, Beloni L, Giannarini L, Sampognaro S, Parronchi P, Manetti R, Annunziato F, Livi C, et al: Progesterone favors the development of human T helper cells producing Th2-type cytokines and promotes both IL-4 production and membrane CD30 expression in established Th1 cell clones. J Immunol 1995;155:128–133.
46 Blois SM, Joachim R, Kandil J, Margni R, Tometten M, Klapp BF, Arck PC: Depletion of CD8+ cells abolishes the pregnancy protective effect of progesterone substitution with dydrogesterone in mice by altering the TH1/TH2 cytokine profile. J Immunol 2004;172:5893–5899.
47 Gibbs RB: Levels of trkA and BDNF mRNA, but not NGF mRNA, fluctuate across the estrous cycle and increase in response to acute hormone replacement. Brain Res 1998;787:259–268.
48 Sohrabji F, Miranda RC, Toran-Allerand CD: Estrogen differentially regulates estrogen and nerve growth factor receptor mRNAs in adult sensory neurons. J Neurosci 1994;14:459–471.
49 Zoubina EV, Fan Q, Smith PG: Variations in uterine innervation during the estrous cycle in rat. J Comp Neurol 1998;397:561–571.
50 Zoubina EV, Mize AL, Alper RH, Smith PG: Acute and chronic estrogen supplementation decreases uterine sympathetic innervation in ovariectomized adult virgin rats. Histol Histopathol 2001;16:989–996.
51 Bjorling DE, Beckman M, Clayton MK, Wang ZY: Modulation of nerve growth factor in peripheral organs by estrogen and progesterone. Neuroscience 2002;110:155–167.
52 Krizsan-Agbas D, Pedchenko T, Hasan W, Smith PG: Oestrogen regulates sympathetic neurite outgrowth by modulating brain derived neurotrophic factor synthesis and release by the rodent uterus. Eur J Neurosci 2003;18:2760–2768.
53 Terness P, Bauer TM, Rose L, Dufter C, Watzlik A, Simon H, Opelz G: Inhibition of allogeneic T cell proliferation by indoleamine 2,3-dioxygenase-expressing dendritic cells: Mediation of suppression by tryptophan metabolites. J Exp Med 2002;196:447–457.
54 Munn DH, Shafizadeh E, Attwood JT, Bondarev I, Pashine A, Mellor v: Inhibition of T cell proliferation by macrophage tryptophan catabolism. J Exp Med 1999;189:1363–1372.
55 Baban B, Chandler P, McCool D, Marshall B, Munn DH, Mellor AL: Indoleamine 2,3-dioxygenase expression is restricted to fetal trophoblast giant cells during murine gestation and is maternal genome specific. J Reprod Immunol 2004;61:67–77.
56 Dong-Ruyl L, Sawada M, Nakano K: Tryptophan and its metabolite, kynurenine, stimulate expression of nerve growth factor in cultured mouse astroglial cells. Neurosci Lett 1998; 244:17–20.
57 Arck PC, Rose M, Hertwig K, Hagen E, Hildebrandt M, Klapp BF: Stress and immune mediators in miscarriage. Hum Reprod 2001;16:1505–1511.
58 Clark DA, Banwatt D, Chaouat G: Stress-triggered abortion in mice prevented by alloimmunization. Am J Reprod Immunol 1993;29:141–147.
59 Foreman JC: Peptides and neurogenic inflammation. Br Med Bull 1987;43:386–400.
60 Stanisz AM, Scicchitano R, Dazin P, Bienenstock J, Payan DG: Distribution of substance P receptors on murine spleen and Peyer's patch T and B cells. J Immunol 1987;139:749–754.
61 Arck PC, Merali FS, Stanisz AM, Stead RH, Chaouat G, Manuel J, ClarkDA: Stress-induced murine abortion associated with substance P-dependent alteration in cytokines in maternal uterine decidua. Biol Reprod 1995;53:814–819.
62 Chaouat G, Zourbas S, Ostojic S, Lappree-Delage G, Dubanchet S, Ledee N, Martal J: A brief review of recent data on some cytokine expressions at the materno-foetal interface which might challenge the classical Th1/Th2 dichotomy. J Reprod Immunol 2002;53:241–256.
63 Aloe L, Bracci-Laudiero L, Alleva E, Lambiase A, Micera A, Tirassa P: Emotional stress induced by parachute jumping enhances blood nerve growth factor levels and the distribution of nerve growth factor receptors in lymphocytes. Proc Natl Acad Sci USA 1994;91:10440–10444.
64 Bonini S, Lambiase A, Bonini S, Levi-Schaffer F, Aloe L: Nerve growth factor: An important molecule in allergic inflammation and tissue remodelling. Int Arch Allergy Immunol 1999; 118:159–162.
65 Braun A, Lommatzsch M, Renz H: The role of neurotrophins in allergic bronchial asthma. Clin Exp Allergy 2000;30:178–186.
66 Burbach GJ, Kim KH, Zivony AS, Kim A, Aranda J, Wright S, Naik SM, Caughman SW, Ansel JC, Armstrong CA: The neurosensory tachykinins substance P and neurokinin A directly induce keratinocyte nerve growth factor. J Invest Dermatol 2001;117:1075–1082.

67 Lindsay RM, Harmar AJ: Nerve growth factor regulates expression of neuropeptide genes in adult sensory neurons. Nature 1989;337:362–364.
68 Toyoda M, Nakamura M, Makino T, Hino T, Kagoura M, Morohashi M: Nerve growth factor and substance P are useful plasma markers of disease activity in atopic dermatitis. Br J Dermatol 2002;147:71–79.

PD Dr. Petra Clara Arck
Biomedizinisches Forschungszentrum, Raum 2.0549, Augustenburger Platz 1
DE–13353 Berlin (Germany), Tel. +49 30 450 553873
Fax +49 30 450 553962, E-Mail petra.arck@charite.de

Markert UR (ed): Immunology of Pregnancy.
Chem Immunol Allergy. Basel, Karger, 2005, vol 89, pp 149–157

The Complement System at the Fetomaternal Interface

Roberta Bulla[a], *Fleur Bossi*[a], *Fabio Fischetti*[b], *Francesco De Seta*[c], *Francesco Tedesco*[a]

[a]Department of Physiology and Pathology, [b]Department of Medicine and Neurology and [c]Department of Reproductive and Developmental Sciences, IRCCS Burlo Garofolo, University of Trieste, Trieste, Italy

Abstract

The placenta has a unique structural organization that allows fetal cells expressing paternal alloantigens to establish a peaceful cohabitation with the maternal immune system. The fetal cells are continuously exposed to the humoral and cellular components of the maternal immune system present in the maternal blood that circulates in the intervillous space and in the decidual vessels. This review deals with the role played by the complement system at the placental level both in physiological and pathological conditions of pregnancies. Complement components found in the placental tissue derive to a large extent from blood circulating in placental vessels. However, some complement components may also be produced locally by macrophages and other cell types. Deposition of complement components at tissue level is usually found in association with inflammatory diseases. This is not the case in placentae in which deposits of complement components can also be documented in physiological conditions not resulting in fetal damage. Protection of the semiallogenic human conceptus against maternal complement activation products is achieved by surface expression of complement regulators that act at different steps of the complement sequence. These complement regulators are localized in a strategic position on the surface of villous trophoblast protecting the fetus from the damage that may derive from uncontrolled complement activation. However, pathological conditions of pregnancies may lead to deposition of a higher amount of complement activation products that may exceed the protection of local complement regulators.

Introduction

The complement system is an important component of innate immunity that contributes to host defense acting either alone or, more often, in collaboration

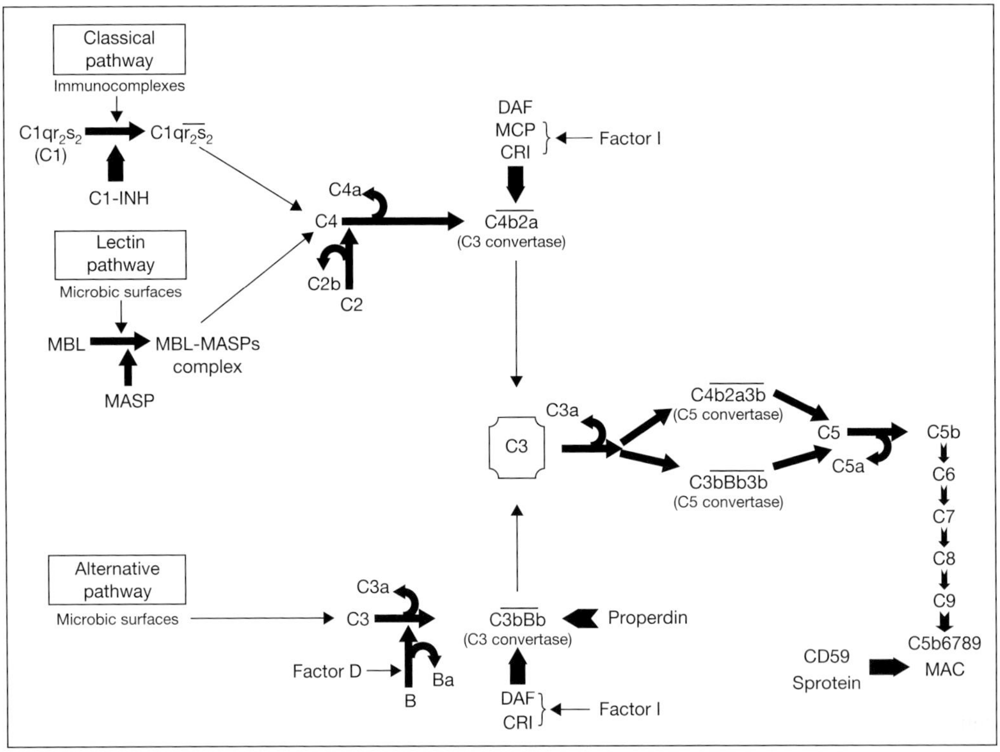

Fig. 1. The complement system. The activation of complement by immunocomplexes (classical pathway), N-acetylglucosamine on the surface of bacterial pathogens (lectin pathway), various activating surfaces such as bacterial cell wall (alternative pathway), the late steps of complement activation and formation of the MAC and principal regulators of complement activation.

with other components of both the innate and acquired immune system. The main function of the complement system is to control infectious agents and to help remove immune complexes and apoptotic cells [1]. The active role of complement in fulfilling this function is ensured by the widespread distribution of complement components in the circulation and in various tissues and also by the multiple biological activities of this system. These activities include opsonization of the target and promotion of inflammation through the recruitment and activation of leukocytes. Although the complement system is organized to distinguish self from nonself, massive activation of complement leads to the release of biologically active products that may cause local damage as a result of a direct cell or tissue destruction or following complement-medi ated leukocyte infiltration. The consequences may be deleterious in all tissues and organs, but become particularly dangerous in organs, like the placenta, the integrity of which is critical for the survival of the fetus.

In this review we describe the organization that the complement system has adopted in the placenta to accomplish its important task of an efficient defense system and to avoid the damaging effect that may derive from an uncontrolled activation of the system.

The placental tissue contains a fully organized complement system that is mostly contributed by the complement components present in the maternal blood circulating in placental vessels, although some components are likely to be produced locally. The conditions for the complement activation at the placental level are essentially similar to those encountered in any other tissue and include immune complexes and infectious agents. However, the placenta is a newly formed organ that undergoes an intense process of tissue remodeling. This inevitably leads to the generation of debris that can activate the complement system resulting in the release of potentially destructive activation products that need to be neutralized.

In humans the developing fetus is not exposed directly to maternal blood except in one specialized organ at the fetomaternal interface, the placenta, the newly formed organ at the uterine level that plays a key role in the maintenance of local tolerance and allows the mother to accept the embryo until completion of pregnancy. The villous trophoblast, the fetal side of the placenta, covers a large surface area of the chorionic villi floating into the intervillous space and forms a continuous barrier that physically separates the mother from the fetus allowing only a selective passage of soluble molecules. The villous trophoblast bearing fetal antigens is continuously exposed to maternal immunocompetent cells present in the blood that circulates in the intervillous space. Syncytiotrophoblast and villous cytotrophoblast have also been found in the maternal circulation and in the lung and provide additional antigenic stimuli of fetal origin for the mother during pregnancy. Trophoblast is not only present on the surface of chorionic villi, but trophoblastic cells are found to be widely diffuse also in the decidua where they contribute to further stimulating the maternal immune system with fetal antigens. Finally, the endovascular trophoblast enters the spiral arteries forming a plug where the arteries open out into the intervillous space and from there these cells move upward replacing the endothelium of the arterial wall [2, 3]. Pregnancy is a unique physiological condition characterized by close physical contact of the maternal immune system with fetal cells expressing paternal alloantigens, which should therefore be recognized as foreign to the mother. The contact between fetal and maternal cells has in general no pathological consequence and does not trigger a maternal immune reaction that leads to fetal death.

The Complement System

The complement system is an effector of nonspecific humoral immunity and it is composed by a group of about 35 proteins either soluble in plasma or associated with cell membranes. The complement proteins are mainly synthesized by several cell types including hepatocytes, monocytes, tissue macrophages, fibroblast, endothelial cells, and adipocytes. Cells from various tissues have also been shown to secrete complement, such as gastrointestinal, urogenital and lung epithelial cells, synoviocytes, and astrocytes. In the genital tract the human endometrium secretes C3 and factor B and the secretion of C3 by rat endometrial epithelial cells appears to be regulated by estrogen [4].

The complement system needs to be activated in order to express lytic and nonlytic activities that are critically important for the host protection from pathogens and other noxious agents. Since inappropriate activation can cause disease, tight regulation of the activation process is required to prevent tissue damage. Complement activation occurs via classical, lectin and alternative pathways. The classical pathway is triggered by immunocomplexes or other nonimmune-activating factors recognized by C1q, which normally circulates in blood as a complex with the two serine protease zymogens, C1r and C1s. [5, 6]. Conversely, the recently described lectin pathway [7, 8] utilizes mannan-binding lectin (MBL) to recognize mannose or N-acetylglucosamine on the surface of bacterial pathogens. The structure of MBL is similar to that of C1q and is normally associated in the blood with the zymogen form of the serine proteases MASP-1 and MASP-2 [9]. These activation pathways share C4 and C2, which are utilized to form the C3 convertase C42. The alternative pathway initiates with the assembly of a C3 convertase on various cellular surfaces, including pathogenic bacteria, parasites, viruses, virus-infected cells and fungi [10]. Factor B, P, D, C3b and the regulators factor I and H are involved in this pathway. Activation of the late components of the complement system from C5 to C9 represents the final step of all three pathways and leads to the assembly of the terminal C complex (TCC). This is the first perforin identified that inserts as membrane attack complex (MAC) into the cell target causing cytolysis [11].

Since the main function of the complement system is to destroy foreign pathogens, it is essential that it is tightly regulated at the key steps of initiation, amplification and membrane attack [12] to avoid tissue injury. The regulator of the initiation step of the classical pathway is the C1-Inh which inactivates C1r and C1s. Other regulators are involved in the regulation of the amplification step. Factor I cleaves C3b/C4b in the presence of cofactor proteins, such as the membrane cofactor protein (MCP), factor H or the complement receptor type 1 (CR1). The decay-accelerating factor (DAF) accelerates the decay of the C3/C5 convertases, while properdin (P) stabilizes the alternative pathway convertase. The lytic activity of MAC is regulated in the fluid phase by clusterin and S protein and on the cell membrane by CD59, which blocks the full assembly of MAC on the host cells.

Deposition of Complement Components on Placentae in Physiological Pregnancies

Deposition of complement components at the tissue level is usually seen in association with diseases. This is not the case with the placenta where deposits of complement components can also be documented in physiological pregnancy. Since trophoblast cells express paternal antigens, these are the cells that can be a potential target of complement-fixing maternal alloantibodies. Syncytiotrophoblast and endovascular trophoblast are in contact with maternal blood and syncytiotrophoblast microvilli embolize into the maternal circulation [13].

The first evidence for the presence of complement at the fetomaternal interface was provided by Faulk et al. [14], who analyzed term and preterm normal human placentae for the presence and distribution of complement components by immunofluorescence and documented deposits of C1q, C4, C5, C6 and C9 in human placenta. These complement components were found to be associated with some stromal cells and areas of fibrinoid necrosis within the trophoblastic mantle and were also seen in the wall of fetal stem vessels. In the case of syncytiotrophoblasts, deposits of these proteins were not seen on the apical plasma membrane but were found to be colocalized with fibrin on trophoblast plasma membranes and perivillous fibrin. Sinha et al. [15] found fluorescence staining C1q in the larger fetal stem vessels of placentae and in stromal cells of chorionic villi. These authors reported a distribution of C4 similar to that observed by Faulk et al. [14] whereas C3d and C9, but not C4, were seen associated with the trophoblast basement membranes. This suggests that the activation pathways leading to complement deposition on trophoblast basement membrane and on perivillous fibrin may be different [15, 16].

Complement components have also been reported to be deposited on spiral arteries in normal pregnancy [17, 18]. Wells et al. [18] analyzed formalin-fixed sections of hysterectomy specimens of normal pregnancies ranging between 4 and 40 weeks of gestational age for the presence of C1q, C3d, C4, C6 and C9. They observed deposits of these components on spiral arteries with the most intense staining for C3d and C9 suggesting that the complement system is likely to be activated through the classical pathway and that a humoral immune response leading to complement activation may be involved in the physiological changes occurring in spiral arteries in the early stage of pregnancy [18].

The TCC represents the end product of complement activation and deposits of this complex can easily be detected using antibodies directed against a neoantigen exposed on the polymerized C9 of the complex, but not on the native molecule. This complex was found to localize in the fibrinoid material of the decidua of the basal plate, in the stroma of the chorionic villi and in the vessel wall of term placentae as subendothelial deposits [19]. The finding of TCC in normal placentae was not unexpected as both early and late complement components are present in term placentae although these studies did not provide conclusive evidence for tissue deposition of the late components in the activated form [19]. TCC deposits did not colocalize with S protein, which is usually associated with the cytolytically inactive complex, indicating that some degree of continuing C activation occurs at the placental level.

The exact mechanism of complement activation leading to deposition of TCC in normal placenta has not yet been clarified. One possibility is that complement is activated by cellular and tissue remnants made available locally by tissue turnover. Mitochondrial membranes, lysosomal enzymes, cytoskeletal intermediate filaments and red blood cell membranes are examples of potential local activators of complement. It is possible that mild deposits of TCC in normal placenta are an expression of a general phenomenon occurring in normal tissue, as they may also be observed in normal human kidney [11].

Regulators of the Complement System in Human Placenta

The protection of the semiallogenic human conceptus against maternal complement activation products is achieved by the surface expression of complement regulators that act at different steps of the complement sequence [20]. The complement regulatory protein DAF or CD55 controls the C3 convertase, while MCP and CR1 are cofactors of the C3b inactivator that cleaves C3b causing degradation of this molecule. CD59, like DAF, is bound to the cell membrane through a GPI anchor and neutralizes the cytolytic activity of the complex inhibiting the polymerization of C9 within the MAC. All these complement regulators are present in placenta from at least 6 weeks of gestation until term.

As a consequence of the direct contact with the maternal blood, syncytiotrophoblast is well protected from complement attack by expressing the three regulatory molecules DAF, MCP and CD59 [21, 22]. In addition, these fetal cells are able to bind S protein or vitronectin, an inhibitor of the terminal complex, from the maternal plasma as a further means of protection [19]. Villous trophoblast expresses very little DAF probably because these cells need less protection from complement attack as compared to syncytiotrophoblast. To demonstrate the protective function of the regulatory molecules, we tested syncytiotrophoblast for its susceptibility to complement-dependent killing using either a complement-fixing antibody-directed syncytiotrophoblast to activate complement through the classical pathway or the cytolytically active MAC in the reactive lysis system [23]. The addition of blocking antibodies to complement inhibitors in both situations resulted in increased cell lysis and the effect was additive when the antibodies were combined in blocking experiments. Interestingly the presence of DAF, MCP and CD59 has also been detected on extravillous trophoblast. We have found that, while CD59 is distributed on all types of trophoblast, DAF and MCP were preferentially expressed on giant decidual cells [24] although these cells are not directly exposed to maternal blood except for the endovascular trophoblast.

The effect of complement on trophoblast is not necessarily cytotoxic and may result either in impairment or in stimulation of the cell function caused by the MAC. It is now well established that the complex formed by the assembly of the five terminal components can be inserted into the membrane of several cell types in a sublytic form exhibiting noncytolytic activity [22].

Complement Deposition on Placentae in Pathological Pregnancies

The role played by complement in the subinvolution of the uteroplacental arteries, a well-recognized cause of hemorrhage in the postpartum period, was investigated by Andrew et al. [25]. Subinvoluted vessels have no endothelial lining whereas uteroplacental arteries normally reendothelialize in the third trimester of pregnancy. Interstitial and occasionally endovascular trophoblast persisted within subinvoluted vessels while these vessels normally reendothelialize during the third trimester so that endovascular trophoblast is not normally present at term. Andrew et al. [26] demonstrated that deposition on C1q, C3d, and C4 was absent in subinvoluted vessels and C9 was detected focally. It is therefore debatable whether vascular complement deposition in abnormal pregnancy is truly immunopathological. Altemani et al. [27] examined placentae with villitis of unknown etiology for the presence and distribution of C1q and C3d and showed the presence of C1q only in the inflamed villi with a diffuse distribution of C1q in the stroma of these villi.

Placentae obtained from preeclamptic patients have been examined for the presence of complement components and complement activation products. These were detected by Sinha et al. [15] in substantial amounts on preeclamptic placentae suggesting that immune processes may be operative in the pathophysiology of this clinical condition. We have extended these observations documenting a marked deposition of TCC both in the decidua and in the villi.

In conclusion, deposition of complement occurs physiologically in placenta indicating that it may be compatible with a physiological progression of pregnancy. It may be involved in the promotion of cell-cell interaction and vascular remodeling. Under these physiological conditions, the presence of complement-regulatory proteins is absolutely essential to protect fetal cells from an uncontrolled activation of the maternal complement. This protection is overcome in pathological situations associated with deposition of a substantial amount of complement activation products.

Acknowledgment

Several authors of this manuscript are members of an European Network of Excellence, entitled 'EMBIC' (Embryo Implantation Control), supported by the European Union (contract no. 512040).

References

1 Fishelson Z, Attali G, Mevorach D: Complement and apoptosis. Mol Immunol 2001;38:207–219.

2 Zhou Y, Fisher SJ, Janatpour M, Genbacev O, Dejana E, Wheelock M, Damsky CH: Human cytotrophoblasts adopt a vascular phenotype as they differentiate. A strategy for successful endovascular invasion? J Clin Invest 1997;99:2139–2151.

3 Damsky CH, Fisher SJ: Trophoblast pseudo-vasculogenesis: Faking it with endothelial adhesion receptors. Curr Opin Cell Biol 1998;10:660–666.

4 Colten HR, Garnier G: Regulation of complement protein gene expression; in Frank M (ed): The Human Complement System in Health and Disease. New York, Dekker, 1998, pp 217–240.

5 Arlaud GJ, Colomb MG, Gagnon J: A novel functional model of the human complement component C1q. Immunol Today 1987;8:106–111.

6 Strang CJ, Siegel RC, Phillips ML, Poon PH, Schumaker VN: Ultrastructure of the first component of human complement: Electron microscopy of the crosslinked complex. Proc Natl Acad Sci USA 1982;79:586–590.

7 Matsushita M, Fujita T: Activation of the classical complement pathway by mannose-binding protein in association with a novel C1s-like serine protease. J Exp Med 1992;176:1497–1502.

8 Ji YH, Fujita T, Hatsuse H, Takahashi A, Matsushita M, Kawakami M: Activation of the C4 and C2 components of complement by a proteinase in serum bactericidal factor, Ra reactive factor. J Immunol 1993;150:571–578.

9 Reid KBM: C1q and mannose-binding lectin; in Volanakis E, Frank M (eds): The Human Complement System in Health and Disease. New York, Dekker, 1998, pp 33–48.

10 Pangburn M, Muller-Eberhard H: The alternative pathway of complement. Semin Immunopathol 1984;7:163–192.

11 Tedesco F, Bulla R, Fischetti F: Terminal complement complex: Regulation of formation and pathophysiological functions; in Szebeni J (ed): The Complement System. Boston, Kluwer Academic Publishers, 2004, pp 97–127.

12 Liszewsi M, Atkinson J: Regulatory proteins of complement; in Volanakis E, Frank M (eds): The Human Complementary System in Health and Disease. New York, Dekker, 1998, pp 9–32.
13 Hamilton WJ, Boyd JD: Specializations of the syncytium of the human chorion. Br Med J 1966; 5502:1501–1506.
14 Faulk WP, Jarret R, Keane M, Johnson PM, Boackle RJ: Immunological studies of human placentae: Complement components in immature and mature chorionic villi. Clin Exp Immunol 1980; 40:299–305.
15 Sinha D, Wells M, Faulk WP: Immunological studies of human placentae: Complement components in pre-eclamptic chorionic villi. Clin Exp Immunol 1984;56:175–184.
16 Vanderpuye OA, Labarrere CA, McIntyre JA: The complement system in human reproduction. Am J Reprod Immunol 1992;27:145–155.
17 Weir PE: Immunofluorescent studies of the uteroplacental arteries in normal pregnancy. Br J Obstet Gynaecol 1981:88:301–307.
18 Wells M, Bennett J, Bulmer JN, Jackson P, Holgate CS: Complement component deposition in uteroplacental (spiral) arteries in normal human pregnancy. J Reprod Immunol 1987;12:125–135.
19 Tedesco F, Radillo O, Candussi G, Nazzaro A, Mollnes TE, Pecorari D: Immunohistochemical detection of terminal complement complex and S protein in normal and pre-eclamptic placentae. Clin Exp Immunol 1990;80:236–240.
20 Harris CL, Morgan BP: The many faces of the membrane regulators of complement; in Szebeni J (ed): The Complement System: Novel Roles in Health and Disease. Boston, Kluwer AcademicPublishers, 2004, pp 129–166.
21 Morgan BP, Holmes CH: Immunology of reproduction: Protecting the placenta. Curr Biol 2000; 10:R381–R383.
22 Nicholson-Weller A, Halperin JA: Membrane signaling by complement C5b-9, the membrane attack complex. Immunol Res 1993;12:244–257.
23 Tedesco F, Narchi G, Radillo O, Meri S, Ferrone S, Betterle C: Susceptibility of human trophoblast to killing by human complement and the role of the complement regulatory proteins. J Immunol 1993;151:1562–1570.
24 Bulla R, Bossi F, Radillo O, de Seta F, Tedesco F: Placental trophoblast and endothelial cells as target of maternal immune response. Autoimmunity 2003;36:11–18.
25 Andrew AC, Bulmer JN, Wells M, Morrison L, Buckley CH: Subinvolution of the uteroplacental arteries in the human placental bed. Histopathology 1989;15:395–405.
26 Andrew A, Bulmer JN, Morrison L, Wells M, Buckley CH: Subinvolution of the uteroplacental arteries: An immunohistochemical study. Int J Gynecol Pathol 1993;12:28–33.
27 Altemani AM, Norato D, Baumel C: Immunological studies in placentas with villitis of unknown etiology: Complement components and immunoglobulins in chorionic villi. J Perinat Med 1992; 20:129–134.

Prof. Francesco Tedesco
Dipartimento di Fisiologia e Patologia, Università di Trieste, via Fleming 22
IT–34127 Trieste (Italy), Tel. +39 040 5584037
Fax +39 040 5584023, E-Mail tedesco@univ.trieste.it

Markert UR (ed): Immunology of Pregnancy.
Chem Immunol Allergy. Basel, Karger, 2005, vol 89, pp 158–168

Asymmetric Antibodies: A Protective Arm in Pregnancy

G. Gutierrez, T. Gentile, S. Miranda, R.A. Margni

IDEHU-Institute of Humoral Immunity Studies (CONICET-UBA),
School of Pharmacy and Biochemistry, University of Buenos Aires,
Buenos Aires, Argentina

Abstract

In normal conditions, a simple change in the pattern of cytokines towards a Th2 response is associated with the production of aggressive antibodies. This fact could not completely explain phenomena such as the fetal survival or the chronicity of certain infections. However, it has been demonstrated that Th2 cytokines increase the proportion of asymmetric antibodies, which are unable to activate effector immune mechanisms (complement fixation, clearance of antigens and phagocytosis). Investigations of asymmetrically glycosylated antibodies demonstrated that these IgG molecules have an extracarbohydrate in one of the Fab regions. This glycosylation affects their antigen interaction turning them into a functionally univalent and blocking antibodies. It has been established that their synthesis is increased under different physiopathological situations involving Th2 responses: chronic infections by extracellular microorganisms, pregnancy and allergic processes. In this review we summarize the experiments performed by our research group over the last years as well as the advances made concerning the role and mechanism of asymmetric antibodies.

The Role of Asymmetric Antibodies

In 1972 we demonstrated in bovine serum albumin (BSA)-inoculated rabbits an immune response characterized by the production of precipitating anti-BSA IgG antibodies, accompanied by 10–20% of IgG antibodies of the same isotype but exhibiting different immunochemical and biological properties [1]. These antibodies lack the ability to fix complement and to form insoluble antigen-antibody complexes and have also been reported in humans and other mammals inoculated with several antigens [2–5]. These IgG molecules have

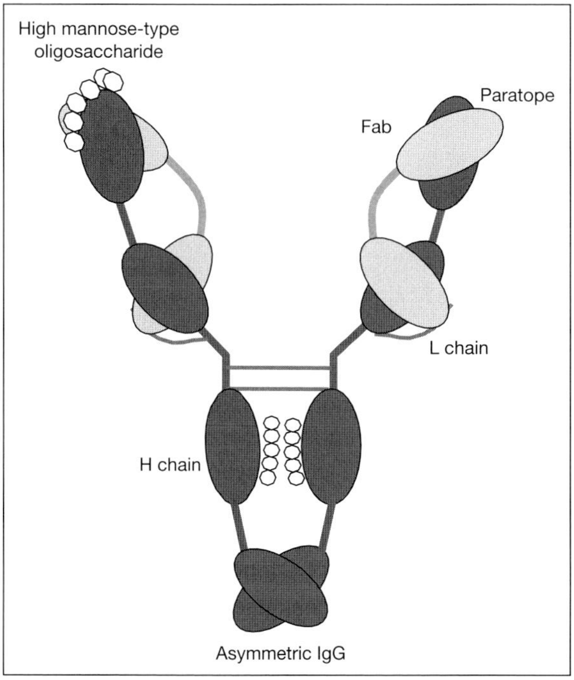

Fig. 1. Asymmetric IgG molecule. One of the Fab fragments is hindered by a high mannose-type oligosaccharide.

two antigen-combining sites of dissimilar affinity: one paratope has a high affinity with a Ko (medium equilibrium affinity association constant) similar to the precipitating antibody, and the other paratope with an affinity for the hapten that is roughly 100 times lower [6]. As a consequence and although they can combine with antigens, they are not capable of triggering immune effector mechanisms. The functional univalence of these antibodies is due to steric hindrance in one of the paratopes due to the presence of an oligosaccharide residue of the high-mannose type, inserted in the Fd fragment of the H chain of one of the Fab regions [7] (fig. 1). Taking this into account, it is possible to isolate these asymmetric IgG molecules from the total IgG present in normal or immune sera using concanavalin A-Sepharose B chromatography [8]. We have demonstrated that a proportion of 10–20% of the IgG molecules in nonimmune sera is asymmetric [9].

Asymmetric IgG antibodies behave as both univalent and blocking ones do. This property enables them to protect the antigen from the aggression by diverse immune mechanisms triggered during the immune response. Therefore, it could be assumed that the existence of these antibodies might be either beneficial or harmful to the host, depending on the 'self' or 'nonself' nature of the antigen. Upon binding self-antigens they could act as protective, regulating antibodies [10]. On the other hand, in certain chronic bacterial and parasitic diseases, the presence of blocking antibodies may favor the evasion mechanisms developed by the pathogen perpetuating the process and leading to chronicity [11].

The percentage of asymmetric antibodies increases in particular situations, for example, following repeated inoculations of particulated antigens and cell suspensions [12]. Asymmetric IgG antibodies react in a competitive manner when they are mixed with precipitating symmetric antibodies of the same specificity, and therefore, the final effect observed will depend on the percentage of each IgG population in the mixture.

By using hybridoma cultures we demonstrated that both symmetric and asymmetric IgG molecules are synthesized by the same clone [13]. Besides, the treatment with endo-N-β-acetylglycosaminidase H, an enzyme that removes oligosaccharides attached to the Asn residue of the protein, transforms the asymmetric IgG into precipitating antibodies, indicating that glycosylation of one of the paratopes of the IgG molecule is a posttranslational phenomenon [7].

Asymmetric Antibodies and Pregnancy

The central role of cytokines in the immune response has been emphasized. It is considered that a Th1-type cytokine profile (IL-2, INF-γ, TNF-α) activates cytotoxic T lymphocytes, whereas a Th2-type cytokine profile (IL-4, IL-5, IL-6, IL-10, IL-11, IL-13) is an inductor of B lymphocytes and noncytotoxic T lymphocytes [14]. It was also postulated that Th1 responses are suppressed during pregnancy; this suppression is accompanied by local expression of Th2 cytokines in placental tissue that may be beneficial for fetal survival [15].

It should be borne in mind that a Th2-type response means antibody production by B cells, and that most of these antibodies, especially those of the IgG class, can fix complement and are involved in other effector immune mechanisms such as phagocytosis and antibody-dependent cell cytotoxicity, among others. Upon binding to antigen epitopes these antibodies trigger the mechanisms that lead to the antigen degradation process. Taking this into account, a change in the cytokine profile involved in Th1- or Th2-type responses could have deleterious effects on the normal course of pregnancy.

In murine pregnancy, antibodies with antipaternal specificity were detected both in serum and fixed on the placenta [16]. These murine antibodies were predominantly of the IgG1 subclass, a non-complement-fixing molecule that can act as a 'facilitating' antibody. Bell and Billington [17] analyzed the participation of the humoral immune response in pregnant females and the predominance of antipaternal blocking IgG antibodies was demonstrated. These findings would indicate that only blocking antibodies, in the context of a Th2-type response, could have an active participation in protection of the fetus during pregnancy. However, in humans and other species, it has been demonstrated that serum antipaternal antibodies having blocking properties are mostly of the same IgG isotypes that usually fix complement.

Considering the antigen-protective properties, asymmetric antibodies could be of importance in the mother-fetus relationship. Studies carried out in our laboratory in 1990 showed that multiparous women, during the first trimester of pregnancy, had a marked increase in asymmetric IgG in serum and that in IgG isolated by 4 *M* KCl treatment of term placenta homogenates the asymmetry percentage reached 60–70%. When the antipaternal lymphocyte activity was investigated by indirect immunofluorescence (IIF) in asymmetric and symmetric IgG isolated from placenta, antibody activity was located in both immunoglobulins, in a 5:1 ratio, indicating the prevalence of asymmetric antibodies in this immune response. We also demonstrated that serum levels of asymmetric IgG decrease after delivery and return to baseline levels within 20–30 days [18].

Even though in primiparous females the increase in asymmetric IgG in serum is moderate and no paternal antilymphocyte antibodies are detected by IIF, this does not mean that the mechanism suggested for multiparous females is not operative in primiparous ones. The cause lies in the sensitivity of the serological method normally used for their detection. An antibody concentration of about 1.5 μg/ml (10^{-8} *M*) or 10^{-11} mol/ml, the sensitivity limit of IIF, multiplied by Avogadro's number (6.2×10^{23}), corresponds to 6×10^{12} molecules/ml or 3×10^{16} molecules in the bloodstream. This number is more than sufficient to block all the possible epitopes present in a human placenta, with a total number of cells calculated to be 10^{12}, each one bearing 10^4 epitopes, not all of which are related to paternal antigens.

The Synthesis of Asymmetric Antibodies and the Placenta

The participation of antipaternal asymmetric IgG antibodies in the maintenance of a successful mother-fetus relationship was demonstrated but the question is how the mechanism of their synthesis is modulated. Considering that the placenta carries out many physiological functions during pregnancy, it was investigated whether the products synthesized by such tissue cells could have some participation in the regulation of the synthesis of those protective antibodies. For this purpose homogenates of human placenta were cultured in RPMI 1640 separating the placental supernatants (PS) after 72 h. Two hybridomas producing different proportions of asymmetric and symmetric IgG1 and IgG2a antibodies, respectively, were supplemented with variable quantities of PS and incubated at 37°C. After 3 days of incubation, the percentage of asymmetric IgG antibodies was determined. A considerable increase in the proportion of these molecules was observed, reaching a peak value of 5–10% PS. When 20% or more PS was added, the proportion of asymmetric IgG antibodies did not increase [19].

These results were confirmed by in vivo studies. Two groups of Fischer rats were inoculated subcutaneously with ovalbumin (OVA) and one of the groups received, prior to inoculations with OVA, several doses of PS by the intraperitoneal route. All animals were bled to determine the percentage of symmetric and asymmetric anti-OVA IgG antibodies. The results obtained showed an increase in the proportion of asymmetric antibodies in animals injected with PS, confirming the results obtained in vitro [20].

In order to isolate and identify the placental factor responsible for the phenomenon described PS from several human placentae from multiparae obtained by cesarean surgery were concentrated and filtered through Sephacryl-200. Several peaks were obtained, their protein concentrations adjusted to the same value and their activities tested by addition to hybridoma 112-B4 (which produces monoclonal anti-DNP antibodies) at different concentrations, followed by evaluation of the proportion of asymmetric anti-DNP IgG antibodies. Several peaks were analyzed, and only a protein peak of a molecular weight of 23–27 kDa was responsible for this effect.

IL-6 and Asymmetric Antibodies

Knowing that IL-6 is associated with the modulation of glycosyltransferase activity by increasing the glycosylation rate of diverse proteins, and that its molecular weight (27 kDa) is similar to that of the protein purified from PS, assays were performed in order to establish whether both IL-6 and the 27-kDa PS fraction were related. In another assay, the 27-kDa protein peak or IL-6 was added to hybridoma cultures. The increase in the proportion of asymmetric IgG antibodies was the same in both cases, displaying maximal efficiency when added at 20 μg/ml (fraction of molecular weight 27 kDa) or 200 U/ml (rhIL-6). This effect was abolished by previous addition of an anti-IL-6 serum to the culture medium or by addition of a high concentration of the 27-kDa fraction or rhIL-6 [21].

Resorption rate of the CBA × DBA/2 murine model usually provides the opportunity to evaluate cytokine influence on the survival of the fetoplacental unit. We demonstrated that at day 9.5 of pregnancy, CBA × DBA/2 fetoplacental units secrete lower IL-6 levels than normal CBA × BALB/c. Although in vitro cytokine production may not reflect accurately the in vivo situation, the present results agree with the hypothesis that CBA × DBA/2 placentae are quantitatively or qualitatively deficient in their production of Th2-type cytokines compared to the non-resorption-prone CBA × BALB/c mating combination. In vivo inoculation of 2,500 U of rhIL-6 was able to increase fetoplacental IL-6 levels up to normal values (CBA × BALB/c fetoplacental IL-6 levels) and this autocrine effect seems to be only local. Moreover, the same dose of rIL-6 was able to decrease the fetal resorption rate as well as to increase the proportion of asymmetric antibodies secreted by placental cells from 6-month-old multiparous CBA × DBA/2 female mice. On the other hand, almost 100% of fetoplacental units were aborted when CBA × DBA/2 females were treated with double doses of rIL-6 (5,000 U) [22].

Furthermore, in normal pregnant women, and in agreement with the same results obtained in animal models, we have also demonstrated an increase in the percentage of asymmetric IgG molecules (38–47%). On the other hand, serum levels in recurrent spontaneous abortion patients were not increased (15–18%). When the recurrent spontaneous abortion women received lymphocyte immunotherapy prior to pregnancy, the serum asymmetric IgG levels increased [23]. These results are consistent with those obtained after repeated inoculations of particulate antigens in rat and rabbit models, where a higher proportion of asymmetric antibodies was found [16, 24].

When analyzing human placental tissues from first-trimester spontaneous abortions, excluding anatomical, endocrinological, chromosomal or infectious etiologies, we observed that syncytiotrophoblast cells expressed high levels of IL-6, and gp80 and gp130 (the two components of IL-6R) [25]. The same observations were also made when we analyzed murine resorption unit cells from a high resorption rate in the CBA/J × DBA/2 mating combination [26].

The above-mentioned studies leave no doubt about the identity of the 27-kDa peak, isolated from human placenta culture supernatants, with IL-6, which is the main responsible factor for the glycosylation of asymmetric IgG molecules, synthesized by the hybridoma. In all likelihood, this is the product that regulates the quality of the humoral immune response during pregnancy, playing a major role in the preservation of the maternofetal relationship. Interleukin regulation of asymmetric IgG synthesis by isolated placenta B cells was also analyzed. In these experiments we showed that the highest increase in asymmetric antibody synthesis was observed when IL-6 was added to placental B lymphocyte cultures in combination with IL-4 and IL-10. Nevertheless, when IL-4 or IL-10 alone or in combination were added to cultures, asymmetric IgG production was not significantly different from unstimulated control cells [27]. In this study we observed that the effect of interleukins on asymmetric IgG synthesis by placental B cells was variable depending upon each cytokine being analyzed separately or in combination.

Some authors have reported that the hormonal microenvironment during pregnancy could contribute to a Th2 response development [28, 29]. In addition, indirect effects of progesterone on in vitro asymmetric antibody synthesis have been shown [30]. The complex expression patterns of interleukins occurring in pregnancy, and even more so, the possible dose-dependent opposite effects of a cytokine and its precise location have been analyzed by Chaouat [31], among others [32, 33].

Intracellular Mechanisms of Asymmetric IgG Glycosylation

Taking into account this evidence the next question to be answered was how does IL-6 modulate an increase in the glycosylation rate of IgG molecules. This glycosylation mechanism takes place during the heavy chain translation in the endoplasmic reticulum of the antibody-producing cells where the UDP-Glc glycoprotein glucosyltransferase (GT), an enzyme involved in the quality control and folding of glycoproteins, participates. In order to analyze modifications in the activity of this enzyme we employed a mouse hybridoma that was cultured in the presence of IL-6 and dexamethasone, two modulators of the asymmetric antibody synthesis. We observed that IL-6 was able to upregulate both the in vitro GT activity and the asymmetric molecule synthesis, while dexamethasone showed an inhibitory effect on both parameters. The correlation analysis between GT activity and asymmetric antibody synthesis found in this in vitro model suggests that GT is involved in the synthesis of asymmetric antibodies. From this bulk of evidence we can hypothesize that IL-6 secreted by trophoblasts and other cell types could promote changes in immunoglobulin H chain folding by modulating GT activity in B lymphocytes, exposing new sequons and facilitating their glycosylation. As a result of this process an increase in antipaternal asymmetric IgG antibodies during gestation is observed [34]. Moreover, we have also demonstrated an enhanced in vitro hsp72 expression induced by IL-6. It is tempting to speculate that hsp72 might act as an intracellular intermediate product in the putative mechanism [35].

According to these results, we have hypothesized that during pregnancy, in the context of a predominant Th2 immune response, where inhibition or no activation of components of the cellular immunity occur, the quality of the IgG antibodies synthesized is modified by IL-6 of placental origin. When the levels of IL-6 secreted by placental cells are low (normal), there is a preferential synthesis of asymmetric glycosylated antibodies, which have a blocking activity and participate in the protection of the fetal antigens against the aggressive biological

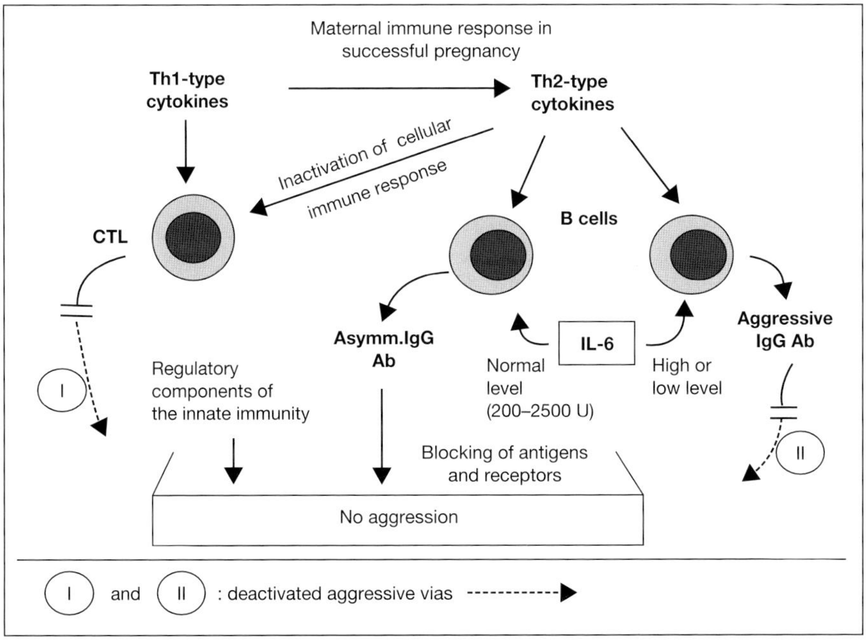

Fig. 2. In a successful pregnancy, the innate immunity participates by inhibiting some aggressive mechanisms. In the adoptive immune response there is a shift in the cytokine profile with the Th2 pattern (IL-4, IL-5, IL-10) predominating over the proinflammatory Th1 cytokines (IL-2, INF-γ, TNF-α) that activate cytotoxic T lymphocytes (CTL), which down-regulates the Th1 response. Furthermore, the Th2 response activates B cells which secrete either aggressor or blocking antibodies depending upon the modulatory effects of the IL-6 secreted by the trophoblast.

mechanisms of the immune response [36]. This could be one of the various mechanisms that facilitate an immunological symbiosis between mother and fetus. Neither lower nor higher levels of IL-6 than the normal ones can enhance the blocking antibody synthesis. Therefore, with an abnormal level of IL-6, there is a predominance of aggressive antibodies (fig. 2).

It was also of interest to evaluate whether the modulation during pregnancy of a humoral immune response with the predominance of asymmetric IgG antibodies was related exclusively to antigens of paternal origin or whether it was a more general phenomenon. To assess this issue, virgin and pregnant Fischer rats were inoculated with OVA. Virgin rats had a normal anti-OVA response, whereas in pregnant rats an increase in the proportion of asymmetric IgG antibodies was observed on day 14 which corresponds to two thirds of the gestation period [20]. Similar results to those obtained in pregnant rats were observed in virgin rats passively transferred with PS. By day 20 postpartum, anti-OVA asymmetric IgG antibodies had decreased to normal levels. These findings indicate that the modulation of an immune response with an increase in the proportion of asymmetric IgG antibodies is a general phenomenon, restricted not only to the antigens of paternal origin, and which ends after delivery with the expulsion of the placenta.

In conclusion, when asymmetric IgG antibodies are specific for self-antigens, they are beneficial to the host, as they can exert regulatory functions. In allergy manifestations, in some autoimmune diseases and especially during pregnancy despite the fact that the antigens responsible for the process are foreign to the host, they also have a beneficial activity. When asymmetric IgG antibodies are specific for the foreign aggressors, as occurs in chronic bacterial and parasitic infections, the predominance of these antibodies proves harmful to the host by blocking the antigens of the pathogen, facilitating its survival and favoring chronicity.

Considering that during pregnancy there is a preferential synthesis of asymmetric IgG antibodies by the mother, whatever the nature of the injected antigen may be, routine vaccination in pregnancy to ensure the transfer of a protective humoral immunity to the fetus is questionable.

References

1 Margni RA, Binaghi RA: Purification and properties of non-precipitating rabbit antibodies. Immunology 1972;22:557–563.

2 Margni RA, Hajos SE: Biological and physicochemical properties of purified anti-DNP guinea pig non-precipitating antibodies. Immunology 1973;24:435–443.

3 Margni RA, Paz CB, Cordal ME: Immunochemical behavior of sheep non-precipitating antibodies isolated by immunoadsorption. Immunochemistry 1974;11:765–770.

4 Cordal ME, Margni RA: Isolation, purification and biological properties of horse precipitating and non-precipitating antibodies. Immunochemistry 1974;11:765–770.

5 Margni RA, Binaghi RA: Non-precipitating asymmetric antibodies. Annu Rev Immunol 1988; 6:534–554.

6 Ronco J, Sciuto E, Leoni J, Margni RA, Binaghi RA: Interaction of purified precipitating and non-precipitating antibodies with hapten and with haptenated protein. Evidence of an asymmetrical antibody molecule. Immunology 1984;52:449–456.

7 Labeta M, Margni RA, Leoni J, Binaghi RA: Structure of asymmetric non-precipitating antibody: Presence of a carbohydrate residue in only one Fab region of the molecule. Immunology 1986; 57:311–317.

8 Leoni J, Labeta M, Margni RA: The asymmetric IgG non-precipitating antibody. Localization of the oligosaccharide involved, by Concanavalin A interaction. Mol Immunol 1986;23:1397–1400.

9 Borel IM, Gentile T, Angelucci J, Margni RA, Binaghi RA: Asymmetrically glycosylated IgG isolated from non-immune human sera. Biochim Biophys Acta 1989;990:162–164.

10 Canellada A, Gentile T, Dokmetjian J, Margni RA: Occurrence, properties and function of asymmetric IgG molecules isolated from non-immune sera. Immunol Invest 2002;31:107–120.

11 Margni RA, Malan Borel I: Paradoxical behavior of asymmetric IgG antibodies. Immunol Rev 1998;163:77–87.

12 Margni RA, Perdigón G, Gentile T, Abatángelo C, Dokmetjian J: IgG precipitating and coprecipitating antibodies in rabbits repeatedly injected with soluble and particulate antigens. Vet Immunol Immunopathol 1986;13:51–61.
13 Morelli L, Leoni J, Fossati CA, Margni RA: Symmetric and asymmetric IgG antibodies are synthesized by the same cellular clone. Mol Immunol 1989;26:789–792.
14 Romagnani S, Parronchi P, Delios MM, Romagnani P, Anunziato F, Piccinni MP, Manetti R, Sampog Movilia C, De Carli M, Maggi E, Del Prete GF: An update on human Th1 and Th2 cells. Int Arch Allergy Immunol 1997;113:153–156.
15 Wegmann TG, Lin H, Guilbert L, Mossmann TR: Bidirectional cytokine interactions in the fetomaternal relationship. Is successful pregnancy a Th2 phenomenon? Immunol Today 1993; 14:353–356.
16 Voisin G, Chaouat G: Demonstration, nature and properties of maternal antibodies fixed on placenta and directed against paternal alloantigens. J Reprod Fertil 1974;21:89–103.
17 Bell SC, Billington WD: Antifetal alloantibody in the pregnant female. Immunol Rev 1983; 75:5–30.
18 Malan Borel I, Gentile T, Angelucci J, Pividori J, Guala MC, Binaghi RA, Margni RA: IgG asymmetric molecules with antipaternal activity isolated from sera and placenta of pregnant woman. J Reprod Immunol 1991;20:129–140.
19 Margni RA, Malan Borel I, Kapovic M, Angelucci J, Miranda S, Kinsky R, Chaouat G: The proportion of symmetric and asymmetric IgG antibody molecules synthesized by a cellular clone (hybridoma) can be regulated by placental culture supernatants. Cell Immunol 1992;142:287–295.
20 Gentile T, Margni RA: IgG asymmetric anti-ovalbumin antibodies synthesized by virgin and pregnant rats. J Reprod Immunol 1995;28:1–13.
21 Gutierrez G, Malan Borel I, Margni RA: The placental regulatory factor involved in the asymmetric IgG antibody synthesis responds to IL-6 features. J Reprod Immunol 2001;49:21–32.
22 Gutierrez G, Sarto A, Berod L, Canellada A, Gentile T, Pasqualini S, Margni RA: Regulation of interleukin-6 fetoplacental levels could be involved in the protective effect of low-molecular-weight heparin treatment on murine spontaneous abortion. Am J Reprod Immunol 2004;51:160–165.
23 Zenclussen AC, Gentile T, Kortebani G, Mazzoli A, Margni RA: Asymmetric antibodies and pregnancy. Am J Reprod Immunol 2001;45:289–294.
24 Gentile T, Malan Borel I, Angelucci J, Miranda S, Margni RA: Preferential synthesis of asymmetric antibodies in rats immunized with paternal particulate antigens. Effect on pregnancy. J Reprod Immunol 1992;22:173–183.
25 Zenclussen AC, Roux ME, Margni RA, Malan Borel I: Interleukin-6 in abortion and in normal placentae histological samples. Placenta 1999;20/5/6:A73.
26 Zenclussen AC, Blois S, Stumpo R, Olmos S, Aria K, Malan Borel I, Roux ME, Margni RA: Murine abortion is associated with enhanced interleukin-6 levels at the feto-maternal interface. Cytokine 2003;24:150–160.
27 Canellada A, Farber A, Zenclussen AC, Gentile T, Dokmetjian J, Keil A, Blois S, Miranda S, Berod L, Gutierrez G, Markert UR, Margni RA: Interleukin regulation of asymmetric antibody synthesized by isolated placental B cells. Am J Reprod Immunol 2002;48:275–282.
28 Piccini MP, Guidizi MG, Biagiotti R, Beloni L, Giannarini F, Livi C, Romagnani S, Maggi E: Progesterone favors the development of human T helper cells producing Th2 type cytokines and promotes both IL-4 production and membrane CD30 expression in established Th1 cell clones. J Immunol 1995;155:128–133.
29 Lim KJH, Odukoya OA, Ajjan RA, Li TC, Weetman AP, Cooke ID: Profile of cytokine mRNA expression in peri-implantation human endometrium. Mol Hum Reprod 1998;4:77–81.
30 Kelemen K, Bognar I, Paal M, Szekeres-Bartho J: A progesterone-induced protein increases the synthesis of asymmetric antibodies. Cell Immunol 1996;167:129–134.
31 Chaouat G: Cytokine networks at the feto-maternal interface: Are the existing paradigms still valid? (abstract MS2–1). Am J Reprod Immunol 2001;46:25.
32 Croy BA: Where now for the Th1/Th2 paradigm of the gestational uterus? J Reprod Immunol 2001;51:1–2.
33 Arck PC, Zenclussen AC, Fest S, Sehmsdorf US, Klapp BF: Challenging the Th1/Th2 dichotomy. Am J Reprod Immunol 2001;45:P11.

34 Miranda S, Canellada A, Gentile T, Margni R: Interleukin-6 and dexamethasone modulate in vitro asymmetric antibody synthesis and UDP-Glc glycoprotien glycosyltransferase activity. J Reprod Immunol, in press.
35 Miranda S, Gentile T, Margni RA: Enhancement of in vitro hsp 72 expression by placental IL-6. Am J Reprod Immunol 2001;46:358–365.
36 Margni RA, Zenclussen AC: During pregnancy, in the context of a Th2-type cytokine profile, serum IL-6 levels might condition the quality of the synthesized antibodies. Am J Reprod Immunol 2001;46:181–187.

G. Gutierrez
Facultad de Farmacia y Bioquímica de la Universidad de Buenos Aires
Junín 956, 4 P.
Buenos Aires 1113 (Argentina), Tel. +54 11 49648260
Fax +54 11 49640024, E-Mail gabgutie@ffyb.uba.ar

In Loving Memory

Professor Ricardo Margni was a well-known and respected Argentinean basic scientist. In 1963, he founded the first Latin-American molecular immunology department at the University of Buenos Aires. He was past chairman of the Institute of Humoral Immunity Studies of the National Council of Scientific and Technical Research and contributed to several studies dealing with immunology of reproduction. He is also the author of books and numerous scientific publications.

In 1970 he discovered asymmetric antibodies and then spent his entire academic life analyzing the impact of these molecules on the success or failure of pregnancy.

He died on December 15, 2004 at the ripe age of 83. He was still working at his lab and sharing his ideas with his colleagues the day before. We will miss him dearly.

Udo R. Markert
Gabriela Gutierrez
Teresa Gentile
Silvia Miranda

Market UR (ed): Immunology of Pregnancy.
Chem Immunol Allergy. Basel, Karger, 2005, vol 89, pp 169–179

Lessons from Reproductive Immunology for Other Fields of Immunology and Clinical Approaches

Udo R. Markert, Justine S. Fitzgerald, Lydia Seyfarth, Joana Heinzelmann, Frauke Varosi, Sandra Voigt, Ekkehard Schleussner, Hans-Joachim Seewald

Department of Obstetrics, Friedrich Schiller University, Jena, Germany

Abstract

Reproduction is indispensable to evolution and, thus, life. Nonetheless, it overcomes common rules known to established life. Immunology of reproduction, and especially the tolerance of two genetically distinct organisms and their fruitful symbiosis, is one of the most imposing paradox of life. Mechanisms, which are physiologically used for induction of said tolerance, are frequently abused by pathogens or tumors intending to escape the host's immune response. Understanding the regulation of immune responses in pregnancy and the invasion of allogeneic fetus-derived trophoblast cells into the decidua may lead to new therapeutic concepts. In transplantation, knowledge concerning local physiological immunotolerance may be useful for the development of new therapies, which do not require a general immune suppression of the patient. In immunological disorders, such as autoimmune diseases or allergies, immune deviations occur which are either prevented during pregnancy or have parallels to pregnancy. Vice versa, lessons from other fields of immunology may also offer new notions for the comprehension of reproductive immunology and may lead to new therapies for the treatment of pregnancy-related problems.

Tumor Immunology

Malignant tumor cells frequently express altered protein patterns which are not recognized as 'self' by the host's immune system [1, 2]. Thus, they are potential targets for immune attacks. A variety of strategies used by tumor cells to escape the host's immune system are similar to those of trophoblast cells.

Immune Escape through Modified Surface Characteristics

To avoid recognition through their tumor-associated antigens, several tumors reduce the expression of classical HLA class I molecules [3]. Instead, many malignant tumors, including melanoma, glioma as well as lymphoproliferative, renal, breast and ovarian cancers, express nonclassical HLA molecules similar to those found in trophoblast cells such as HLA-G, soluble HLA-G (sHLA-G) or HLA-E [4–6]. This provides an advantage over tumor cells within the same tumor, which do not express these molecules [7]. The introduction of classical HLA I molecules into deficient tumor cells enhances T cell responses [8]. Several tumors downregulate the expression of costimulatory molecules, such as CD80 or CD86, a phenomenon also seen in trophoblast cells. In these cases also, the introduction of the lacking molecules induces T cell responses [8, 9]. Furthermore, the costimulatory molecule B7-H1 induces apoptosis in activated T cells and is expressed in high concentrations on syncytiotrophoblast, cytotrophoblast and various tumors [9, 10].

Immune Modulations via Soluble Substances

Trophoblast cells express a wide spectrum of soluble factors to modify the immune response of the host. These include, besides sHLA-G, a multitude of others, the tryptophan-catabolizing and T cell-inactivating enzyme indoleamine dioxygenase (IDO) and hormones such as β-human choriogonadotropin [11–13]. These factors are also expressed by a number of nontrophoblastic tumors [11, 13]. Furthermore, progesterone induces the production of an immunomodulatory blocking factor in lymphocytes, and adequately coined progesterone-induced blocking factor (PIBF) [14, 15]. PIBF is also released by numerous tumors and can serve as a diagnostic tumor marker in most body fluids [16].

Invasion

Trophoblast cells display potent invasive capacities. The expression of several matrix metalloproteinases is protooncogene regulated and allows for their invasive expansion into the maternal host tissue [17]. Most tumors use similar enzymes for invasion [18]. Regulation and intracellular signaling are also similar for trophoblast invasion and tumors, as can be recognized in the invasion-promoting role of signal transducer and activator of transcription-3 (STAT3), a regulatory molecule found in both several tumors, but also trophoblast cells [19–22].

Pregnancy-Malignancy Interactions

Malignant diseases and pregnancy may occur simultaneously, but this is a very rare event. The frequency was 0.32/1,000 deliveries in an US American retrospective study analyzing the coexistence of cancer and pregnancy between

1974 and 2002 in Chicago, Ill. All cancer patients had healthy babies [23]. Another study reports 3,500 annual cases of such a coexistence in the United States, which is equivalent to 1/1,000 deliveries [24]. The most frequently occurring tumors are breast cancer (1/3,000 deliveries), cervical cancer (1.2/10,000 deliveries), malignant melanoma (frequency unclear) and lymphomas (1–6/6,000 deliveries). Generally, pregnancy and cancer do not affect each other. Cytostatic cancer therapies are tolerated by mature fetuses and therapeutic abortions are extremely seldom. Vertical transmission of cancer to the conceptus is extremely rare and is up to 30% caused by melanoma and less frequently by leukemias, and breast and lung carcinomas [24].

Microbiological Immunology

Parasites

Parasites need to survive in a xenogeneic ambience. Extracellular parasites, especially helminths, have developed some escape mechanisms similar to those of the conceptus. They are able to suppress inflammatory cytokines of Th1 and Th2 type [e.g. IL-2, IL-5 and interferon-γ (IFN-γ)] in the host comparable to pregnancy [25]. In contrast to pregnancy though, helminths usually induce a strong increase of IgE production, but without atopic symptoms [26]. The underlying mechanisms seem to occur beyond the classical Th1-Th2 concept and may be regulated by IL-10 producing innate effector and regulatory T cells, a phenomenon which is also observed in pregnancy [27–29]. Intracellular parasites, such as Leishmania, also use similar mechanisms. They live within dendritic cells, from where they induce T cells to produce IL-4, IL-5 and IL-10 [30]. This expression correlates with their persistence, whereas induction of IFN-γ leads to their elimination [30].

Viruses

Viruses live intracellularly and need to protect their host cells from immune attacks for a certain time span. Such an attack would release the virus and make it a potential target for the host's immune system. Many viruses implement this requirement by downregulation or modification of HLA expression on host cells. This is most efficient, when they avoid presentation of virus particles to cytotoxic T cells, but without activation of innate immune responses through NK cells. For this aim, several viruses induce HLA I profiles similar to those on trophoblast cells. The human cytomegalovirus downregulates surface expression of most HLA isotypes, but not for HLA-C, HLA-E and HLA-G. In the same manner, the human immunodeficiency virus and the human herpes virus 8 suppress HLA expression, except for HLA-C and HLA-E in both cases.

These findings are consistent with the role of HLA-C, HLA-E and HLA-G on trophoblast cells for escaping innate immune responses [31].

Pregnancy-Infection Interactions

All infections are principally possible during pregnancy. Generally, the maternal immune system responds similarly to that of nonpregnant individuals during pregnancy, but a few exceptions exist. Infections during pregnancy have several aspects. Generalized effects of infections, such as fever, weakness, gastrointestinal problems and malnutrition, may disturb pregnancy greatly, but not directly due to immune reactions. Especially in cases of reproductive tract infection, the placenta or fetus may be involved or harmed, possibly triggering premature contractions or deliveries. Placental infections may lead to placental damage associated with loss of function, release of inflammatory mediators, induction of premature labor and subsequent preterm birth and transplacental infection of the fetus [32]. In some cases, the immune response against the germ may also activate decidual immune cells to work against the maintenance of pregnancy. For example, abortions occur in mice infected with *Leishmania maior*, when the parasite is rejected, while pregnancy supports survival of the parasite [30, 33].

Transplantation

Rejection Mechanisms

Allogeneic transplantations of many organs and tissues are a routine method in medicine. Without supplemental treatments transplants would be rejected. Nonself proteins, and especially allogeneic HLA molecules are highly immunogenic and capable of generating severe immune reactions in the host which lead to rejection. Mainly cytotoxic T cells, T helper cells and NK cells, but also all other immune cells of the host are involved in rejections [34].

Antirejection Therapies

It is necessary to suppress expected immune responses in order to avoid rejections. The optimal requirements of drugs are to protect the graft maximally while affecting the host's immune system minimally so that susceptibility for infections and tumors might be avoided. Pregnancy offers an almost perfect model of a graft being tolerated locally by the immune system while simultaneously only marginally limiting general immunity. Factors which protect the fetus may denote the potential for future drugs in immunosuppressive therapies of transplantation patients.

Similar to the presence of protective antibodies in pregnancy, such as BA11 or asymmetric antibodies, the application of alloantibodies prior to transplantation prolongs graft survival in mice, but the mechanisms of their action are unclear [35–37].

Recent studies indicate a capacity of IDO, a main player for maternofetal tolerance in pregnancy, to protect graft in allograft transplantation among rats [38].

Pregnancy-Transplantation Interactions

Pregnancy is, with very few exceptions of liver insufficiency, a strict contraindication for transplantation. Transplantations accidentally performed during pregnancy are extremely seldom. Both successful and nonsuccessful transplantations with different pregnancy outcomes are reported. It can be assumed that cases of failure are mostly not published and occur at a higher frequency than reported in the literature. The high-dose application of immunosuppressive drugs may lead to a loss of control of trophoblast invasion and disturb several fundamental functions of decidual immune cells. One case of a hydatidiform mole following renal transplantation in early pregnancy is reported and may have been related to such a loss of invasion control [39].

Cases of pregnancy several months or years after transplantation are much more frequent and often successful. Doses of immunosuppression are much lower than shortly after transplantation and, therefore, better tolerable. Thus, pregnancy is not a strict contraindication for transplant patients anymore [40].

Autoimmune Diseases

Loss of Tolerance

Mechanisms of self-tolerance and tolerance against the semiallogeneic fetus are regulated on different levels. Self-tolerance is mainly induced through T cell selection and depletion in the thymus, whereas tolerance to fetal cells is a peripheral event. Thus, the reasons for a loss of tolerance against self-antigens initiating an autoimmune disease and against nonself antigens are manifold and mostly distinct.

Immunosuppressive Therapy

Nonetheless, knowledge of the physiological tolerance of the fetus may lead to the development of therapeutic strategies for treatment of autoimmune diseases that do not require a general suppression of the immune system, especially in the case of organ-specific reactions. The problems are similar to those of therapies following transplantation. The above-mentioned pregnancy-supporting

IDO is currently under successful experimental investigation in animal models for therapeutic approaches to induce tolerance in autoimmune diseases, such as diabetes or autoimmune encephalomyelitis [41, 42].

Pregnancy-Autoimmune Disorder Interactions

Pregnancies in women with autoimmune diseases are generally risky, but the risk depends very much on the type of disease, localization, activity, severity and necessary treatment. Reasons for complications in pregnancy may be due in a large part to nonimmunological problems of the disease, such as liver or kidney insufficiency. The activation of the immune system in autoimmune disorders is frequently accompanied by a Th1-dominated cytokine imbalance which may be disturbing pregnancy, it being a Th2-related period. In up to 50% of couples with recurrent pregnancy loss, antiphospholipid antibodies are present, but the causal association is unclear [43].

Frequently, the state of autoimmune diseases changes during pregnancy [44]. For example, rheumatoid arthritis improves in more than 70% of patients, which is associated with maternal-fetal disparity in alleles of HLA-DRβ1, DQα and DQβ [45, 46]. However, the course of systemic lupus erythematosus is more variable. Highly specific autoantibody profiles in the mother are related to neonatal lupus syndromes with congenital heart block as the most severe one [45].

The immunosuppressive treatment of autoimmune diseases that may not be abandoned during pregnancy in order to maintain vital organ functions may fundamentally disturb the decidual immune balance, induce preterm labor or affect the development of the fetal immune system [47]. A meta-analysis indicated a non-significantly increased prevalence of preterm birth in patients with cyclosporine therapy during pregnancy, but the reasons seem to be multifactorial [48].

Initiation of autoimmune diseases during pregnancy is very seldom, but the prevalence of most autoimmune diseases is higher in women with children compared to those without. In several recent studies, cells of fetal origin were detected in inflamed foci of autoimmune diseases many years after pregnancy and such microchimerism was interpreted as a possible inducer of the reaction [49, 50].

Allergies

The Th2-Prone Immune Response

Similar to pregnancy, allergies occur with a Th2-favored cytokine profile. In their case, IgE production is induced as was described above for certain parasites and in contrast to pregnancy. However, distinct from parasite-induced IgE, allergies induce a specific production [26]. These differences may be due to distinct costimulatory signals joining the cytokine signals from T helper cells to B cells, such as CD154-CD40 interactions, which occur in allergies, but are not observed in the placenta or during pregnancy [51, 52].

Fetal Programming for Allergies

Allergies are multifactorially induced diseases. Several patterns of circumstances, which may favor the development of allergies, are described. One fragment of such patterns is the hereditary component with more detailed observations revealing that maternal allergies were a stronger factor than paternal allergies. This finding led to the conclusion that allergic events during pregnancy may increase the risk of allergies in later life. Subsequent mouse model experiments supported these hypotheses [53, 54].

Immunotherapies in Allergy

Immunotherapies in allergy may induce a cytokine shift towards Th1, which is mostly well known and accepted for insect venom immunotherapies. To avoid the risk of negative interference with the Th2-favored pregnancy, immunotherapies should not be initiated during pregnancy. If a patient on a well-tolerated maintenance dose of immunotherapy becomes pregnant, immunotherapy can be continued. Although insect venom immunotherapy is the strongest Th1 inducer and poses the highest risk for pregnancy, it represents an exception and may be initiated during pregnancy, because a sting may be a life-threatening event. This risk can only be lowered by immunotherapy and should be initiated in highly allergic pregnant women, although the induction of premature events may be possible. Several cases of abortions have been reported under such circumstances [55]. Therefore, all aspects of risks versus benefits must be weighed very carefully.

The IDO Concept

IDO also seems to display a potential for allergy treatment. Ovalbumin-induced allergic asthma in mice could be inhibited by application of IDO [56]. Patients with asymptomatic atopy display increased IDO activity compared to symptomatic individuals, indicating a major role for the regulation of the clinical state of allergy [57].

Pregnancy-Allergy Interactions

Allergy is a frequent disease and coexistence with pregnancy occurs commonly. Very severe symptoms, such as anaphylaxis, severe asthma or generalized dermatitis may harm pregnancy and the fetus due to organ dysfunction rather than to the underlying immune disorder itself. The most common complications of asthmatic women during pregnancy are meconium-stained amniotic fluid, preterm labor or delivery, oligohydramnios, and pregnancy-induced hypertension [58]. Necessary immunomodulatory or immunosuppressive treatment may also affect the decidual immune balance or impair growth and development of the fetus [58]. It is not yet clear to what extent decidual mast cells or other immune cells are involved in allergic reactions and if they significantly release mediators inducing premature labor or delivery in humans. In animal models such events were induced experimentally [59, 60]. In conclusion, it should be recommended that allergic mothers avoid allergens during pregnancy or, better, to treat allergies by immunotherapy before pregnancy.

Concluding Remarks

Immunology of reproduction includes a wide span of physiological immune reactions and modulations, which allow and support the development of the semiallogeneic fetus. Many of them are also used by a variety of non-pregnancy-related pathologies.

The better understanding of these immunological features will be helpful for both the treatment of fertility disorders as well as the treatment of numerous diseases facilitated through modifying immune responses.

Thus far, several discoveries in the field of reproductive immunology, such as the role of the Th1/Th2 balance, HLA-G, IDO or PIBF, offered new concepts for general immunology. There is no doubt that further lessons will follow.

Acknowledgment

Several authors of this manuscript are members of an European Network of Excellence, entitled "EMBIC" (Embryo Implantation Control), supported by the European Union (contract no. 512040).

References

1 Novellino L, Castelli C, Parmiani G: A listing of human tumor antigens recognized by T cells: March 2004 update. Cancer Immunol Immunother 2005;54:187–207.
2 Kawakami Y, Fujita T, Matsuzaki Y, Sakurai T, Tsukamoto M, Toda M, Sumimoto H: Identification of human tumor antigens and its implications for diagnosis and treatment of cancer. Cancer Sci 2004;95:784–791.
3 Chang CC, Campoli M, Ferrone S: HLA class I defects in malignant lesions: What have we learned? Keio J Med 2003;52:220–229.
4 Amiot L, Le Friec G, Sebti Y, Drenou B, Pangault C, Guilloux V, Leleu X, Bernard M, Facon T, Fauchet R: HLA-G and lymphoproliferative disorders. Semin Cancer Biol 2003;13:379–385.
5 Rebmann V, Regel J, Stolke D, Grosse-Wilde H: Secretion of sHLA-G molecules in malignancies. Semin Cancer Biol 2003;13:371–377.

6 Bukur J, Seliger B: The role of HLA-G for protection of human renal cell-carcinoma cells from immune-mediated lysis: Implications for immunotherapies. Semin Cancer Biol 2003;13:353–359.
7 Algarra I, Garcia-Lora A, Cabrera T, Ruiz-Cabello F, Garrido F: The selection of tumor variants with altered expression of classical and nonclassical MHC class I molecules: Implications for tumor immune escape. Cancer Immunol Immunother 2004;53:904–910.
8 Koc S, Kather A, Markert UR, Durst M, Schneider A, Kaufmann AM: Enhancement of immunogenicity of Jeg3 cells by ectopic expression of HLA-A*0201 and CD80. Am J Reprod Immunol 2003;50:243–253.
9 Petroff MG, Chen L, Phillips TA, Azzola D, Sedlmayr P, Hunt JS: B7 family molecules are favorably positioned at the human maternal-fetal interface. Biol Reprod 2003;68:1496–1504.
10 Dong H, Chen L: B7-H1 pathway and its role in the evasion of tumor immunity. J Mol Med 2003; 81:281–287.
11 Mellor AL, Munn DH: IDO expression by dendritic cells: Tolerance and tryptophan catabolism. Nat Rev Immunol 2004;4:762–774.
12 Malek A, Sager R, Willi A, Muller J, Hanggi W, Leiser R, Bersinger N: Production of protein hormones by cultured trophoblast cells isolated from term and early placentae. Am J Reprod Immunol 2000;43:278–284.
13 Stenman UH, Alfthan H, Hotakainen K: Human chorionic gonadotropin in cancer. Clin Biochem 2004;37:549–561.
14 Szekeres-Bartho J, Varga P, Pejtsik B: ELISA test for the detection of an immunological blocking factor in human pregnancy serum. J Reprod Immunol 1989;16:19–29.
15 Szekeres-Bartho J, Polgar B, Kozma N, Miko E, Par G, Szereday L, Barakonyi A, Palkovics T, Papp O, Varga P: Progesterone-dependent immunomodulation. Chem Immunol Allergy. Basel, Karger, 2005, vol 89, pp 118–125.
16 Lachmann M, Gelbmann D, Kalman E, Polgar B, Buschle M, Von Gabain A, Szekeres-Bartho J, Nagy E: PIBF (progesterone induced blocking factor) is overexpressed in highly proliferating cells and associated with the centrosome. Int J Cancer 2004;112:51–60.
17 Bischof P, Truong K, Campana A: Regulation of trophoblastic gelatinases by proto-oncogenes. Placenta 2003;24:155–163.
18 Davidson B, Reich R, Risberg B, Nesland JM: The biological role and regulation of matrix metalloproteinases (MMP) in cancer. Arkh Patol 2002;64:47–53.
19 Knöfler M, Sooranna SK, Daoud G, Whitley GS, Markert UR, Xia Y, Cantiello H, Hauguel-de Mouzon S: Trophoblast signalling: Knowns and unknowns – A workshop report. Placenta 2005; 26:549–551.
20 Corvinus FM, Fitzgerald JS, Friedrich K, Markert UR: Evidence for a correlation between trophoblast invasiveness and STAT3 activity. Am J Reprod Immunol 2003;50:316–321.
21 Poehlmann TG, FJ, Meissner A, Wengenmayer T, Friedrich K, Markert UR: Trophoblast invasion: Tuning through LIF, signalling via Stat 3. Placenta 2005;26:537–541.
22 Fitzgerald JS, Tsareva SA, Poehlmann TG, Berod L, Meissner A, Corvinus FM, Wiederanders B, Pfitzner E, Markert UR, Friedrich K: Leukemia inhibitory factor triggers activation of Signal Transducer and Activator of Transcription 3, proliferation, invasiveness, and altered protease expression in choriocarcinoma cells. Int J Biochem Cell Biol, in press.
23 Jacobs IA, Chang CK, Salti GI: Coexistence of pregnancy and cancer. Am Surg 2004; 70:1025–1029.
24 Pavlidis NA: Coexistence of pregnancy and malignancy. Oncologist 2002;7:279–287.
25 Maizels RM, Balic A, Gomez-Escobar N, Nair M, Taylor MD, Allen JE: Helminth parasites – masters of regulation. Immunol Rev 2004;201:89–116.
26 Yazdanbakhsh M, van den Biggelaar A, Maizels RM: Th2 responses without atopy: Immunoregulation in chronic helminth infections and reduced allergic disease. Trends Immunol 2001;22:372–377.
27 Hesse M, Piccirillo CA, Belkaid Y, Prufer J, Mentink-Kane M, Leusink M, Cheever AW, Shevach EM, Wynn TA: The pathogenesis of schistosomiasis is controlled by cooperating IL-10-producing innate effector and regulatory T cells. J Immunol 2004;172:3157–3166.
28 Heikkinen J, Mottonen M, Alanen A, Lassila O: Phenotypic characterization of regulatory T cells in the human decidua. Clin Exp Immunol 2004;136:373–378.

29 Aluvihare VR, Kallikourdis M, Betz AG: Tolerance, suppression and the fetal allograft. J Mol Med 2005;83/2:88–96.
30 Krishnan L, Guilbert LJ, Russell AS, Wegmann TG, Mosmann TR, Belosevic M: Pregnancy impairs resistance of C57BL/6 mice to *Leishmania major* infection and causes decreased antigen-specific IFN-gamma response and increased production of T helper 2 cytokines. J Immunol 1996; 156:644–652.
31 Huddleston H, Schust DJ: Immune interactions at the maternal-fetal interface: A focus on antigen presentation. Am J Reprod Immunol 2004;51:283–289.
32 Redline RW: Placental inflammation. Semin Neonatol 2004;9:265–274.
33 Krishnan L, Guilbert LJ, Wegmann TG, Belosevic M, Mosmann TR: T helper 1 response against *Leishmania major* in pregnant C57BL/6 mice increases implantation failure and fetal resorptions. Correlation with increased IFN-gamma and TNF and reduced IL-10 production by placental cells. J Immunol 1996;156:653–662.
34 Rocha PN, Plumb TJ, Crowley SD, Coffman TM: Effector mechanisms in transplant rejection. Immunol Rev 2003;196:51–64.
35 Jalali GR, Arck P, Surridge S, Markert U, Chaouat G, Clark DA, Underwood JL, Mowbray JF: Immunosuppressive properties of monoclonal antibodies and human polyclonal alloantibodies to the R80K protein of trophoblast. Am J Reprod Immunol 1996;36:129–134.
36 Oluwole SF, Tezuka K, Wasfie T, Stegall MD, Reemtsma K, Hardy MA: Humoral immunity in allograft rejection. The role of cytotoxic alloantibody in hyperacute rejection and enhancement of rat cardiac allografts. Transplantation 1989;48:751–755.
37 Gutierrez G, Gentile T, Miranda S, Margni RA: Asymmetric antibodies: A protective arm in pregnancy. Chem Immunol Allergy. Basel, Karger, 2005, vol 89, pp 158–168.
38 Bauer TM, Jiga LP, Chuang JJ, Randazzo M, Opelz G, Terness P: Studying the immunosuppressive role of indoleamine 2,3-dioxygenase: Tryptophan metabolites suppress rat allogeneic T-cell responses in vitro and in vivo. Transpl Int 2005;18:95–100.
39 Markert UR, Klemm A, Flossmann E, Werner W, Sperschneider H, Funfstuck R: Renal transplantation in early pregnancy with acute graft rejection and development of a hydatidiform mole. Clin Nephrol 1998;49:391–392.
40 Mastrobattista JM, Katz AR: Pregnancy after organ transplant. Obstet Gynecol Clin North Am 2004;31:415–428, vii.
41 Grohmann U, Fallarino F, Bianchi R, Orabona C, Vacca C, Fioretti MC, Puccetti P: A defect in tryptophan catabolism impairs tolerance in nonobese diabetic mice. J Exp Med 2003; 198:153–160.
42 Sakurai K, Zou JP, Tschetter JR, Ward JM, Shearer GM: Effect of indoleamine 2,3-dioxygenase on induction of experimental autoimmune encephalomyelitis. J Neuroimmunol 2002;129:186–196.
43 Group TECW: Physiopathological determinants of human infertility. Hum Reprod Update 2002; 8:435–447.
44 Elenkov IJ, Chrousos GP: Stress hormones, proinflammatory and antiinflammatory cytokines, and autoimmunity. Ann NY Acad Sci 2002;966:290–303.
45 Buyon JP: The effects of pregnancy on autoimmune diseases. J Leukoc Biol 1998;63:281–287.
46 Nelson JL, Hughes KA, Smith AG, Nisperos BB, Branchaud AM, Hansen JA: Remission of rheumatoid arthritis during pregnancy and maternal-fetal class II alloantigen disparity. Am J Reprod Immunol 1992;28:226–227.
47 Ostensen ME, Skomsvoll JF: Anti-inflammatory pharmacotherapy during pregnancy. Expert Opin Pharmacother 2004;5:571–580.
48 Bar Oz B, Hackman R, Einarson T, Koren G: Pregnancy outcome after cyclosporine therapy during pregnancy: A meta-analysis. Transplantation 2001;71:1051–1055.
49 Kolialexi A, Tsangaris GT, Antsaklis A, Mavroua A: Rapid clearance of fetal cells from maternal circulation after delivery. Ann NY Acad Sci 2004;1022:113–118.
50 Nelson JL: Microchimerism and autoimmune disease. N Engl J Med 1998;338:1224–1225.
51 Phillips TA, Ni J, Hunt JS: Cell-specific expression of B lymphocyte (APRIL, BLyS)- and Th2 (CD30L/CD153)-promoting tumor necrosis factor superfamily ligands in human placentas. J Leukoc Biol 2003;74:81–87.

52 Markert UR, Bar C, Niess JH, Vogelsang H, Zwacka G: Elevated CD154 (CD40 ligand) synthesis in T-cells from allergic patients after nonspecific stimulation in vitro. J Investig Allergol Clin Immunol 1999;9:248–252.
53 Uthoff H, Spenner A, Reckelkamm W, Ahrens B, Wolk G, Hackler R, Hardung F, Schaefer J, Scheffold A, Renz H, Herz U: Critical role of preconceptional immunization for protective and nonpathological specific immunity in murine neonates. J Immunol 2003;171:3485–3492.
54 Herz U, Joachim R, Ahrens B, Scheffold A, Radbruch A, Renz H: Allergic sensitization and allergen exposure during pregnancy favor the development of atopy in the neonate. Int Arch Allergy Immunol 2001;124:193–196.
55 Markert UR, Arck PC, Peiker G, Mock BA: Might wasp venom desensitization induced Th2 to Th1 shift cause pregnancy failure? Am J Reprod Immunol 2002;47:193–195.
56 Hayashi T, Beck L, Rossetto C, Gong X, Takikawa O, Takabayashi K, Broide DH, Carson DA, Raz E: Inhibition of experimental asthma by indoleamine 2,3-dioxygenase. J Clin Invest 2004; 114:270–279.
57 von Bubnoff D, Fimmers R, Bogdanow M, Matz H, Koch S, Bieber T: Asymptomatic atopy is associated with increased indoleamine 2,3-dioxygenase activity and interleukin-10 production during seasonal allergen exposure. Clin Exp Allergy 2004;34:1056–1063.
58 Beckmann CA: The effects of asthma on pregnancy and perinatal outcomes. J Asthma 2003; 40:171–180.
59 Bytautiene E, Romero R, Vedernikov YP, El-Zeky F, Saade GR, Garfield RE: Induction of premature labor and delivery by allergic reaction and prevention by histamine H1 receptor antagonist. Am J Obstet Gynecol 2004;191:1356–1361.
60 Bytautiene E, Vedernikov YP, Saade GR, Romero R, Garfield RE: Degranulation of uterine mast cell modifies contractility of isolated myometrium from pregnant women. Am J Obstet Gynecol 2004;191:1705–1710.

PD. Dr. Udo R. Markert
Abteilung für Geburtshilfe, Friedrich-Schiller-Universität
DE–07740 Jena (Germany), Tel. +49 3641 933763
Fax +49 3641 933764, E-Mail markert@med.uni-jena.de

Author Index

Subject Index